MORE BOOKS FROM THE SAGER GROUP

The Swamp: Deceit and Corruption in the CIA
An Elizabeth Petrov Thriller (Book 1)
by Jeff Grant

Chains of Nobility: Brotherhood of the Mamluks (Book 1-3)
by Brad Graft

Meeting Mozart: A Novel Drawn from the Secret Diaries of Lorenzo Da Ponte
by Howard Jay Smith

Death Came Swiftly: A Novel About the Tay Bridge Disaster of 1879
by Bill Abrams

A Boy and His Dog in Hell: And Other Stories
by Mike Sager

Miss Havilland: A Novel
by Gay Daly

The Orphan's Daughter: A Novel
by Jan Cherubin

Lifeboat No. 8: Surviving the Titanic
by Elizabeth Kaye

Hunting Marlon Brando: A True Story by Mike Sager

See our entire library at TheSagerGroup.net

LIVING BEYOND NORMAL
AN AUTISTIC AUTOBIOGRAPHY

ADAM A.F. SHERMAN

Living Beyond Normal: An Autistic Autobiography

Copyright © 2022 Adam A. F. Sherman

All rights reserved.

No part of this publication may be reproduced, stored in a retrieval system, or transmitted, in any form or by any means, electronic, mechanical, photocopying, recording, or otherwise, without the prior written permission of the publisher.

Published in the United States of America.

Cover and Interior Designed by Siori Kitajima, PatternBased.com

Cataloging-in-Publication data for this book is available from the Library of Congress.

ISBN-13:
eBook: 978-1-950154-96-8
Paperback: 978-1-950154-97-5

Published by The Sager Group LLC
(TheSagerGroup.net)

LIVING BEYOND NORMAL
AN AUTISTIC AUTOBIOGRAPHY

ADAM A.F. SHERMAN

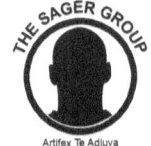

CONTENTS

Chapter 1: The Spotlight 1

Stage One: Birth to Adolescence 5
Chapter 2: A Clean Slate 7
Chapter 3: First Stage is Denial.. 13
The Declassified Psychiatry Files of Adam A.F. Sherman 17
Chapter 4: On the Surface 31
Chapter 5: Bloody Knuckles and Bold-Faced Lies 35
Chapter 6: Escalation at Its Finest 41
Chapter 7: Empires Fall 45
Chapter 8: Despair and Deserted Islands 49
Interlude: Reflection and Self-Introspection 59
Chapter 9: Salvation Lies Within 63

Stage Two: Young Adulthood 71
Chapter 10: It Follows 73
Chapter 11: The First Step 79
Chapter 12: Phoenix Rising 83
Chapter 13: Peak Sensation 89
Chapter 14: Curveballs and Conundrums 95
Chapter 15: A Crazy Twisted Thing Called Love 105
Interlude II: Impressions and the Little Things 109
Chapter 16: Hopes, Dreams, and High Notes 113

Stage Three: Adulthood 121
Chapter 17: Crashing from the High 123
Chapter 18: Sticks and Stones with Smoke and Mirrors 131
Chapter 19: A Brief Respite and a Return to Madness 141
Interlude III: Responsibility, Regret and Acceptance 149
Chapter 20: Learning to Breathe Again 153
Chapter 21: One Door Closes 161

Chapter 22: Another Door Opens 169
Chapter 23: Welcome to the Family 173
Chapter 24: Parts in the Sum of the Whole 179
Chapter 25: Closing the Book to Adventure 191
Chapter 26: There Is No End, Only New Beginnings 197

Acknowledgements 203
About the Author 210
About the Publisher 211

CHAPTER 1
THE SPOTLIGHT

"In a time of universal deceit, telling the truth is a revolutionary act." — George Orwell

The street is wide and empty, the hot Florida sun beating down on a quiet, North Miami neighborhood, reflecting off the pavement, the cars, the fences, and shining onto a young man in a gray short-sleeved shirt and light blue jeans wandering down the lane, lost in the depths of his mind, in the joy of his own world, just him and the little toy truck he has in his hand. His imagination has created a world where this big rig is rolling down the road; whether it is in the city streets or the open road is not known, nor is it known if he is driving the truck or imagining himself willing the truck to move on its own. Whatever the fantasy is, he only has his mind's eye and real eyes for his toy and the world he has created. He has drifted down the road for a short while, not focused on where he is, not paying attention to anything but his toy, and completely oblivious to the trouble that an overzealous onlooker in that neighborhood has in store for him.

Everything happens at once. The fantasy and his focused attention to the toy vanishes as a middle-aged African American male in a light green short-sleeved shirt and dark shorts suddenly appears and asks him to come back to the facility he has apparently left, then several police cars suddenly appear in the street the two are standing in, policemen jumping out of their cars, blocking all exits and training their standard-issue Glock 19 pistols and a sniper rifle at them, demanding that these two normal-looking, casually dressed men get down on the ground and drop their "weapons." The older man lies down on his back with his hands up in the air, while the young man sits in the middle of the street, shaking and clutching his toy truck for dear life, quivering in fear of the numerous men in dark uniforms ready to use their trigger fingers. The man lying down continuously yells to the police that he is behavioral therapist Charles Kinsey and that the young man, Arnaldo Soto, is his autistic patient from a special needs group home. He repeatedly insists that they have no weapons and that the "gun" is just a toy truck.

The feeling in Kinsey's leg is at first like an insect bite, but then the pain rushes in and the blood begins to run into the street like rain into a gutter as he realizes he has been shot. The police rush in and promptly handcuff an injured and severely pained Kinsey, along with a traumatized Soto, confiscating his toy in the process. They are taken into custody and Kinsey is rushed to a local hospital. On the surface, the events of that day look like another racially charged shooting of an unarmed African American male that the Black Lives Matter movement would quickly pick up and show to the world to foment new protests and action against the police department. It later emerges, however, that the policeman holding the sniper rifle was trying to shoot Soto, for he believed that the toy was a gun, as reported by a 911 call claiming a "suicidal man with a gun" was pacing the streets, and Kinsey subsequently ended up as collateral damage.

This story that I watched on the headline news in the summer of 2016 is one of many that plague the world of those who are struggling with social disorders and other developmental disabilities. It does not matter whether the condition is minor or severe, for every single affected individual has a story to tell, whether it is the disabled reporter that then-presidential candidate Donald Trump mocked on national television or the autistic boy who was so noisy that a "concerned parent" wrote a hateful letter to the boy's family telling them to either move or euthanize the child. The stigma on mental illness and disorders is all too real and pervasive in our everyday lives, and when this stigma turns into hate or a misunderstanding gone very wrong, the unthinkable can happen and those who have no control over their suffering end up being victims of their own circumstances.

We as a people have come a long way over the course of human history, but no matter how advanced or progressive our social development has been, in every society there are always issues, people, and even whole communities that are overlooked and neglected. The disabled and socially challenged community is no exception, and it includes upward of sixty million people worldwide suffering from various forms of autism. It has most often been shunned by the spotlight, while the issues of race, homophobia, politics, international relations, and economic disparity triumph in attention given and treatment received. The Reverend Martin Luther King Jr., one of my childhood heroes, once said, "injustice anywhere is a threat to justice everywhere." For too long, a great many people, those considered part of the disenfranchised, have been mistreated well into postmodern history, and despite major efforts and progress throughout the past century, disparity, ignorance, and hate continue to ripple beneath the surface. Even with those living in the shadows of society, such devolved feelings, actions, and/or lack thereof have caused significant damage on a personal level as well as to society, and as such, allow for those who are victimized to continue suffering in silence.

These issues have not gone unnoticed, and yet they have not been prioritized either. The media has a habit of passing over important stories and focusing more on negativity rather than the positive actions that address the problems we face in this modern era. It has not stopped individuals and organizations from fighting to bring these issues and the communities affected by them to the forefront, yet general ambivalence, if not outright apathy toward the disabled, socially challenged, and mentally ill continues unabated. Just as there is still de facto racism and homophobia in the world, so too are there many people who view this community as less than human, as individuals who get what they deserve.

The world cannot be completely rid of hate, as much as many of us (*especially me*) would like to believe, but it also cannot be allowed to stand by and permit the continued proliferation of ambivalence and antagonism. Nor can it be allowed to cultivate a culture where people grow up looking down on others who are different or unable to develop like their normal human counterparts. Every human being on this planet has something to contribute and is every bit as deserving of acceptance, love, friendship, and camaraderie, and the fight to realize that dream and make it a reality continues on. Every person from the disabled and socially challenged community has a story to tell, and none of those stories are more important than another, for they are all equally deserving of attention from the public. While this story is of one individual and may be different from others' stories, it also shares similarities and highlights about how we are all connected and how not a single one of us is ever truly alone.

I am a person with autism. I am not a hero, I am not an activist, and I am not special; I am just a person who is doing what I believe is the right thing to do. I hope that this benefits those who are like me, as well as people with other internal struggles of their own. I also want those considered neurotypical ("*normal*") to know that we are here, that we are as much a part of the human race, and that we deserve acceptance, understanding, and love. I am my own unique person, yet I also have many traits and abilities that put me in the worlds of both neurotypicals and those with autism. Autism itself is a spectrum: just like the colors of the rainbow, no two autistic people are the same in their development, and yet they share similar behaviors that put them into the same category.

From my earliest stage of memory to the present day, this narrative will chronicle the effects of being touched by autism and the events that resulted from interactions that were made, and continue to be made, as life progresses. From victory to defeat, through adversity and inclusion, and to rock bottom and back up again, the aim of this story will be to show that despite profound differences, I, like so many others, am also the same as most people in this world. I am here to do right by others and contribute to the unity we have in our humanity and our drive to move forward and achieve our dreams together.

STAGE ONE

BIRTH TO ADOLESCENCE

"Within the core of each of us is the child we once were. This child constitutes the foundation of what we have become, who we are, and what we will be."

— Neuroscientist Dr. Rhawn Joseph

CHAPTER 2
A CLEAN SLATE

The darkness turned into light the morning I was born in a Catholic hospital in the center of Tokyo, Japan. The light became figures of the midwife, the nurses, the doctor, and my parents. The figures became the surroundings that were the delivery room where I was weighed to make sure I was healthy enough to go home. Finally, the surroundings expanded to include a wide expanse of city blocks and green parks as my parents took me home for the first time. The blank void that was the beginning of my life had begun to fill, even if I have no memory of it. With a memory like mine that stretches back to some of my earliest days, I still have to count on the memories and stories of my parents, some of which are too embarrassing to say aloud. As far as they were concerned, apart from a couple of occasions—such as when a family friend visiting us in Hawaii observed that, for a two-year-old, I was as Zen as the Dalai Lama—I lived a normal toddler's life.

Inheritance begins from birth, when you get your mother's eyes or when you like dogs the way your father does, but it goes deeper than that as you grow up, and I can say that in many ways I am like my parents, who are the most perfectly odd couple I have ever known. How they met is defined as a tale of two oddballs: my father was the youngest of four siblings and came from a long line of New York–based Jewish ancestors dating back to the 1860s when they emigrated from Poland, Ukraine and Hungary, while my mother was the second of four siblings in a Catholic family consisting of a German World War II survivor mother and a German-Irish American father who was a US Air Force colonel and served in the Vietnam War. My mother's family moved constantly to many different military bases throughout America and occasionally to countries such as Turkey and Japan, while the only move my father's family made was from New York to Los Angeles when he was ten years old. Their time as teenagers continued as stark contrasts: my father became laid back and go-with-the-flow as he let his hair grow out, took up basket-weaving in high school, and grew into the hippie counterculture movement; my mother attended Catholic schools where the nuns beat with rulers the students who stepped out of line. Later, in public high school, and as editor of her school's newspaper, her standout moment was writing an article critical of the principal's conduct. Initially, she was expelled, though widespread media coverage pressured the school into readmitting her. Eventually the laid-back hippie met the rebellious Catholic at the start of his first year and her second year at the University of California, Santa Cruz, and for cosmic reasons I will never truly comprehend, they fell in love.

The beginning of what has become forty-five years of "togetherness" and counting started with their completing their degrees in American studies and moving to San Francisco together. My mother started a job with United Press International, and my father worked in a bookshop while waiting for his big break, which came when my mother went to Hastings Law School and referred him to UPI for her same job. Despite my mother's law degree, my parents decided to embark on a sojourn into journalism, and so began many years of accomplishments that felt like something out of the beloved classic film *Forrest Gump*, where just like the titular character, my parents had no shortage of adventures when it came to the places they went, the stories they found, and the people they met. My father would speak to me of the time when he had tea with Supreme Court Justice Thurgood Marshall and how he interviewed Robert F. Kennedy's assassin at his first parole hearing; my mother told of how she bumped into Arnold Schwarzenegger at a gym in South Korea during the 1988 Summer Olympics and interviewed him on a whim and how she worked alongside Harvey Milk on a presidential campaign before he became a famous politician. Their work eventually took them to Asia, where my mother worked in Japan, and my father in South Korea and other nearby countries. Eventually, they both worked for NHK, Japan's largest broadcasting corporation. At that time, they decided to make their then-sixteen years together official, so they married at the US embassy in Tokyo, which also happened to be when my mother was eight months pregnant with me.

When opposites attract in the way my parents have, you get an overt sense of what their behaviors and personalities are like, along with what was learned and passed down to me. As far back as I can remember, my parents have been kind, compassionate, and loving to me and my younger brother Nicholas (*Nick, as he prefers to be called*). However, in certain situations, their reactions would be quite different: my mother would often be quick to assert herself and be the first to mete out discipline if, for example, we refused to do our chores, while my father would more often act calmly and try to find a fitting solution to this and other household problems. When there was the need to entice my brother and me to find hobbies and be productive, my mother would step in and offer numerous options for us to pick from (*sometimes with the threat of picking for us if we couldn't make up our minds*), such as violin lessons, martial arts classes, or acting courses, while my father supported her but also believed that we would find an interest on our own due to our curious natures. The mixing of such opposing personalities (*my mother's Type A, anxiety-laced mental drive; my father's cool, diplomatic, Type B approach*) confused and sometimes upset me growing up, often because I did not know which was the right position to believe and take, and resulted in me being at odds with my mother's assertiveness at times and feeling more comfortable around my father because of his more passive nature. Despite these differences, there has never been any question that they have loved me with all of their hearts, and that having my mother's diligence and developing my father's Zen spirit in me is an inheritance I treasure.

Zen was the first description of me, and the next description has stuck with me to this day: encyclopedic. Memory and vocabulary are talents I have possessed and been aware of since the age of three. Every person, every place, anything read or spoken, and any event that has made an impression on me is truly lasting as far as my recall is concerned. The earliest memory I have is when I was in daycare at the Temple Emanu-El synagogue in San Francisco, playing with a friend who also shared my first name (*we would meet again eleven years later in middle school in the East Bay Area, where I would recognize him despite how long it had been*) and waiting in a classroom for my father to come and pick me up. I also have partial memories about being taken care of by a nanny who was from Israel, and how my parents looked so reassured when trusting her with my life. My father would tell me years later that he felt comforted knowing that she knew how to break down and refit an Uzi submachine gun just for fun.

The combination of growing up, having a predisposition for solid memory recall and showing natural talent for certain subjects and activities brings to mind another fancy phrase from my growing vocabulary: *tabula rasa*. In both philosophy and psychology circles, it is an idea that describes how we are born without built-in mental content and that our development and knowledge comes from experience and perception. It was always a given that I was learning new things in school, from my parents, friends, and other figures I met as I matured. I believed this was normal for any child in society. However, I often wondered why I had certain abilities that left other people impressed. I remember at the age of ten when I was visiting an aquarium and, due to my fascination with animals, essentially took over the job of the guide because of what I was able to remember, despite not having read a book on those aquatic animals in several years. While my parents later informed me that the staff was amazed with my vast knowledge, they also noticed how the guide herself was shocked that a kid had shown her up on the tour. Being that young and having always been encouraged to embrace my talents, I quickly shrugged the encounter off and continued as I was.

From about the age of three to fourteen, my attitude about life was what one would call a glass completely full. I always saw the best in people no matter what the situation or the content of character, was always willing to make friends wherever I could, and was open to learning new things, such as martial arts and studying geology while hiking in the hills around the Napa Valley. Since my family and I moved around every few years because of my parents' wanderlust journalism careers (*from Japan to Hawaii to Lake Tahoe, Napa, and finally the San Francisco Bay*), I brought this curiosity and positive mode of thinking with me wherever I went. My parents were the kind of people who wanted me to have as wide a perspective as possible. They would take my brother and me on trips abroad every year, teach us about our mixed Jewish/Catholic backgrounds, and pay homage through various religious holidays, mostly Hanukkah and Christmas. Most importantly, they taught us to learn to respect ourselves and exercise free will and choice in a careful, considerate, and respectful manner so that we could better respect others and feel in control of our futures.

They never forced us to go to church or synagogue or fraternize with specific people of their choosing, as that did not mesh with their belief in us being free, independent thinkers with a right to choose, despite my mom having been made to attend church and religious schooling when she was a child. Having that level of freedom allowed me to fully express myself the way I wanted, helped me feel confident in school by earning good grades and never voluntarily missing a day of education, and inspired me to participate in various events for a number of causes, such as running laps to raise money for the impoverished. Through this I generated a strong belief that anything I start, I need to finish, whether it was a class project or fulfilling a promise I made to someone. My life at that stage was heading in the right direction; I had everything I wanted, and anything else that came along for the right reasons I would gladly accept, because, as far as I believed, the life my parents wanted for me, and the life I was slowly shaping for myself, was coming to fruition.

With every triumph, however, there were always problems to deal with, the earliest of which I can remember came at age eleven. I was stuck in two worlds, one where girls are considered "icky" and had "cooties," and the other where you begin to realize that there is a nascent degree of attraction. One girl, K.P. seemed to be in the same quandary as me, and she acted on it by asking me to a school dance. She was exceptionally tall for her age, standing the same five foot four inches that I was at the time, with long, flowing brown hair, a mild assortment of freckles across her face, piercing blue eyes, curved eyebrows, and a playful, slightly teasing smile. Being a horse riding enthusiast, she wore skin tight jeans, cowgirl boots, and a flannel jacket over a white short-sleeved shirt. Curious as I was, I accepted her invitation and tried to spend time with her. All too quickly, it went wrong. First came the avoidance, where she would look at me strangely, followed by a quick walk into the women's restroom. Next came the various other strange looks she would give me, from looks of surprise quickly followed by dismissive ones to those of complete disgust.

K.P. eventually took to her cruelest action of all, manipulating me to inadvertently and unwittingly participate in a scheme involving the escalation of a feud she was having with an erstwhile best friend. While promising to be my date to the school dance, she had me disinvite her former friend from a major birthday party she was throwing for herself. Having never been prepared for a situation of manipulation and acting off of my attraction to her, I went through with it. As a result, I experienced what would be the first of many feelings of remorse and regret when our fifth grade teacher discovered the deception. Thankfully, I was cleared of wrongdoing and then treated as a pawn and victim of her scheme as well. From there, K.P. escalated her negative behavior toward me, calling me names and accusing me of being something I had never heard before, but I would learn all too well later on in life: a stalker. Her erratic behavior —from initial attraction and kindness to high-strung cruelty and viciousness—confused and upset me to no end and made me question if I even knew and understood the people I was growing up with. Being a kid, of course, I ended up quickly shrugging off these insecurities, and with other people still treating me well, I continued on with being the same person I was. No one ever believed the accusations against me, and K.P. was disciplined for it as well as for what she did to her former friend, but the result of my actions and the pain they caused, unbeknownst to me, would be a harbinger of worse events to come, events that would challenge my perspective on who I was, how I was raised, and if I even knew myself at all.

CHAPTER 3
FIRST STAGE IS DENIAL

Flash-forward: Three years later

I should have seen it coming. This cannot be real. This is not me; I refuse to believe this is me. Three sentences, three meanings; when someone says that they should have seen it coming, the most common context for me is someone describing the loss of an important high school basketball championship, a long-term relationship gone bad, or lamenting the passing of an older relative. In hindsight, I should have seen it coming: the various, inexplicable trips to the strange doctors I had never met before and often never saw again, the times I was pulled out of class and sent to see the therapist and other school administrators, my parents never explaining why I had to see so many "experts" whose fields I knew nothing about. The one question I kept asking every time I met with these people: "why have I been asked to see you and why am I being interrupted from school for no apparent reason?" Each time, I never got more than a vague response about how it was "standard procedure" and cleared by my parents.

When someone says something is not real, a painful feeling usually accompanies that statement of denial, whether it is horrific events brought to life on the news or the receiving of distressing, personal news too difficult to bear. For me, it started with being pulled out of class again and out of school for the entire day. For once, I was quiet, not questioning my parents as I had done countless times before, watching the towns, marshlands, and sections of the San Francisco Bay pass by out the car window as we headed south toward the town of Santa Clara. We soon pulled into the parking lot of a medical clinic, where my parents handed me off to a couple of middle-aged female psychiatrists who took me into a large room.

The difference between this room and the others I had been in was staggering. The walls were covered in what looked like soundproof padding, the splotchy black and white tiles on the floor matched those of my middle school multi-purpose room, and there was a small table in the middle of the room with some random toys and board games, along with two chairs. One of the psychiatrists excused herself from the room, and the other sat down with me at the table. As I sat, I noticed something on the wall to the immediate right, which I had first mistaken as a mirror; it quickly became apparent, especially after all of my watching of procedural dramas, that it was actually a two-way mirror, and when I got close, I could make out the shapes of three people I quickly deduced were my parents and the psychiatrist who had stepped out. It also became apparent to me that I had been put into something that resembled an interrogation room, with my parents playing the part of police monitoring my behavior and answers and the psychiatrist in front of me asking questions like an investigator. The questions were nothing new, mostly asking about my interests, my friends, and how I saw the world around me. In a way, it was less painful than I thought, and better than the times as a little kid when I was asked to imitate what I thought were strange movements (demonstrating an arm flap, mirroring their movements, etc.) and to obey commands (staying silent and solving complex puzzles in certain amounts of time, answering random questions at light speed without thinking first, etc.) for things I did not understand. All the while, I wondered that out of all the random visits to these doctors and "specialists" throughout the last ten years of my life, why was this one so important that my parents had to sit behind a pane of glass and watch me?

When someone says this is not me and refuses to believe it, it is often considered in the context of rejecting the perception of those around them, thereby compounding a sense of denial. Furthermore, it could also mean that some factual discovery has been made, one considered to be upsetting to the person about to be informed, setting the stage for denial. Informed is exactly what it was for me, as I was eventually led out of the room and into a conference hall with a long table, where my parents and several more psychiatrists and medical professionals were seated. A sense of dread like I had never known filled me: This felt worse than being brought to the principal's office in the third grade for play-fighting like Power Rangers. This felt like a sentencing in court, but for what? What did I do? What would warrant such a cloak and dagger medical approach throughout my life that resulted in my fourteen-year-old self being made to sit in front of some grim-looking officials?

The news was delivered swiftly and matter-of-factly: After much study throughout my life, they had concluded that my official diagnosis was autism, also known as Asperger's syndrome. The shock of this news made me zone out; I barely heard or paid attention to anything they were telling me, as a range of emotions were coursing through my system—anger mixed with shame, sadness with depression, shock with amplified anxiety—all from being told I was not a normal kid. As it turned out, they were describing symptoms that included an increase in stress, anxiety, and depression (in my case situational depression, not the clinical type where there is no reason for depression that randomly appears). They went on to describe how they observed that I did not notice nonverbal cues on their faces; how my fidgeting, ultra-observant traits for everything outside of social signs, and impulsive tendencies classified as atypical human behavior; and how once I started describing something, I was completely focused on it and compelled to finish without noticing the changes and flow of conversation and social atmosphere constantly metamorphosing around me. They then attempted to reassure me that it was not that bad, as I was "lightly" touched by autism and did not exhibit more serious symptoms like an inability to communicate, constant stress over keeping routine or breaking it, or even having extremely narrow interests in subjects and life. Their assurances meant nothing to me, as I still felt a metaphoric train running over me from the news of my now-confirmed condition, the realization that my parents misled me about all past doctor visits, and how I went from feeling like a normal, functioning kid to something I knew the more ignorant people back home would label me in so many derogatory terms, freak being the "nicest" one.

The journey back home was not as quiet as when it began, for I was deaf to all but the sense of betrayal I felt from my parents, the wave of shock that was continuing to batter me senseless, and the rapid building of a wall that would become the unmoving, unceasing representation of my denial. All too quickly, I declared that we were never to speak of this again, that no one, not even Nick, would ever know what transpired in that clinic, and that from now on, I was to be treated as a "normal" kid and that any mention of autism was taboo and forbidden, or else the consequences to them would be nothing short of severe.

[Disclaimer: I will not use the term Asperger's syndrome from this point forward because of my research that resulted in the discovery that the man the syndrome was named after, Dr. Hans Asperger, did his research and practice in cooperation with the Nazis in the Greater German Reich and knowingly sent two disabled children to their deaths at a euthanasia center, that I know of. Furthermore, in 2013 the American Psychiatry Association removed Asperger's syndrome from the Diagnostic and Statistical Manual for Mental Disorders (DSM) and replaced it with Autism Spectrum Disorder]

THE DECLASSIFIED PSYCHIATRY FILES OF ADAM A.F. SHERMAN

(*Note*: These are only assessments of my behavior and mannerisms from ages five, nine, and fourteen, and are in no way a true reflection of who I am as a person, only what was observed at the time. Some information has been redacted due to irrelevance and privacy concerns.)

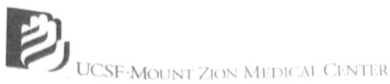
UCSF-MOUNT ZION MEDICAL CENTER

DIVISION OF BEHAVIORAL AND
DEVELOPMENTAL PEDIATRICS

September 17, 1997

J. Lane Tanner, M.D.
Interim Director
415-353-7766
Fax 415-353-9532

Re: Adam Sherman
DOB: 11/26/91
Age: 5 Years, 9 Months
Unit #: 331 03 26-3 7251
DBDP #: 97-169

CONFIDENTIAL
TO BE RELEASED
ONLY WITH PERMISSION OF THE
DIVISION OF BEHAVIORAL AND
DEVELOPMENTAL PEDIATRICS

EARLY CHILDHOOD CLINIC SUMMARY LETTER

As a diagnostic team, we determined that the DSM-IV diagnosis of Asperger's Syndrome was appropriate.

The social reciprocity aspect of the his difficulties is an indicator of the type of disorder which Adam appears to have. The results of the Autism Rating Scale that looked at the relationships, emotional responses, body use, adaptation to change, listening and visual responses, fear and nervousness -- as well as other responses -- were completed with a borderline score for Adam at the junction of non-autistic with mild-moderately autistic.

Adam is less impaired than many autistic children but his dysfunction in social interaction and his restricted interests and intake of information is considered significant enough to place him in the Asperger's category. He does not have all of the characteristics of Asperger's, but he does meet the criteria by having several of the characteristics. The characteristics he has include a qualitative impairment in social interaction, as manifested by the following two areas: 1) marked impairment in the use of multiple nonverbal behaviors, such as eye-to-eye gaze, facial expression, body postures and gestures to regular social interaction; and 2) failure to develop peer relationships appropriate to his developmental level. He also shows a restricted behavior and interest in activities, as manifested by an inflexible adherence to specific nonfunctional routines and preoccupation with restricted pattern of interests that is not typical of his age because of his intensity and focus. We believe that although Adam does not fit each of the qualifying descriptives in this disorder, he does have enough descriptors to meet the criteria. He is a high functioning child with good intellectual potential and the prognosis for change through growth is considered good.

Kathleen Peters, Ed.D.
Licensed Educational Psychologist
Nationally Certified School Psychologist
Licensed Marriage, Family, Child Counselor
Assistant Clinical Professor

KP/rd

cc: Parents
    Medical Records

(ecc\sherman.kp)

Name: Adam Sherman
Date of Birth: 11/21/91
Age at Testing: 9 years, 11 months
Handedness: right
Dates Tested: 11/06/01; 11/20/01

SUMMARY

In summary, Adam Sherman is a right-handed, 9-year, 11 month-old youngster referred for neuropsychological testing at the request of Russell Reiff, M.D., a behavioral-developmental pediatrician at Kaiser San Francisco. The current assessment was requested in order to evaluate Adam's current diagnostic and neurocognitive status. Adam lives at home with his parents and 6-year-old brother and is attending 4th grade at Vichy Elementary School.

Adam's birth, perinatal and developmental histories are unremarkable. There is no known history of problems in the prenatal period. His parents recall that his developmental milestones were "generally delayed slightly". There is no outstanding medical history, with the exception of multiple ear infections and a tonsillectomy and adnoidectomy two years ago for obstructive sleep apnea. Hearing tests to date have been normal Adam's younger brother has a history of unexplained hypotonia, but has responded well to physical therapy.

Although Adam's parents describe him as having a "warm heart and "enthusiasm for friends and family, they are also concerned about his social and communication skills, and difficulties with lack of flexibility, a tendency to become frustrated and angry when dealing with new situations, rigid thinking and poor organizational skills.

An assessment done at the UCSF-Mt. Zion Early Childhood Clinic when Adam was 5-years, 9-months old found a nonverbal IQ of 109 on the Leiter International Performance Scale. His verbal reasoning skills, expressive language and visual motor integration skills were described as falling within the low average range. Mild to moderated delays were noted in pragmatic language skills and qualitative impairments were describe in social interaction and in Adam's behavior and range of interests.

A recent evaluation done by the Napa County SELPA showed academic achievement ranging from the low average to the bottom of the superior range. Adam gave his best performance on a test of spelling to dictation and had the most difficulty on subtests assessing understanding of written material and a written composition. Borderline impairments in visual-motor integration and motor control were seen, with superior visual-perceptual skills. In addition, the school district evaluation documented relative weaknesses in reading comprehension in comparison to reading decoding skills, as well as between math computation as opposed to math reasoning skills.

The neuropsychological assessment described in this report appears to offer a reasonably valid and reliable estimate of Adam's current level of functioning. Despite problems with impulsivity and evidence of frustration when faced with challenging novel tasks, Adam typically put forth a good amount of effort. He showed no difficulty understanding what was being asked of him, and there were no apparent gross perceptual or motor problems were interfering with his ability to perform. However, Adam demonstrated a mild motor tic characterized by a slight sideways jerking of his head that seemed to occur at times of slight stress.

Overall, Adam's performance on cognitive testing (the WISC-III) places him in the low average range (FIQ=88). A statistically and clinically significant differences was seen between verbal and nonverbal functioning (VIQ=101; PIQ=77). Differences of this magnitude occurred in only 6% of children in the standardization sample. A statistically and clinically significant discrepancy was also seen between Adam's mildly impaired performance on tests assessing visual processing speed and his average performance on tests assessing ability to attend to simple auditory information (FD=104; PS=75). Discrepancies of this size or larger were seen in 7.5% of the standardization sample.

Mild impairments were also seen in Adam's performance on WISC-III subtests assessing visual-spatial and visual-constructional skills and on a test of social judgement and commonsense (Block Design and Comprehension). In contrast, Adam gave his best performance on a subtest that assesses factual knowledge about the world (Information), where he scored in the superior range. No significant differences were seen between Adam's performance on academic testing done by the school district and his current scores on tests of intellectual ability.

Despite average to above average functioning on tests of basic perception, attention and language, Adam demonstrated significant deficits in many aspects of complex, higher order mental functioning. In particular, moderate to severe impairments were seen in both verbal and nonverbal abstract and conceptual reasoning, as well as in overall cognitive flexibility. Adam showed a strong tendency to become stimulus bound, or to have great difficulty perceiving more than a single salient aspect of a task, word or image.

Adam typically performed in the average range on tests assessing the ability to attend to a single stimulus (i.e. strings of digits, sounds, pictures or words). However, he demonstrated borderline to mild impairments on tasks that required him to shift his attention flexibly between competing stimuli. This finding is consistent with the pattern of deficits seen on tests assessing cognitive flexibility.

Memory testing revealed a relative weakness in immediate memory, although his performance tended to improve with the passage of time. This suggests that Adam needs more time to consolidate new information than do most people. In addition, Adam showed a pattern of mild to moderate impairment in immediate recall of visual/nonverbal information. Although his performance improved over a delay when asked to recall relatively noncomplex information, he continued to show moderate impairments when asked to recall complex visual information after a 30-minute delay. An analysis of his performance revealed considerable difficulties in organizing complex novel visual information for effective storage and retrieval.

Some inconsistencies were seen in Adam's functioning on tests of motor speed and strength. Adam demonstrated an unusual pattern of nondominant hand superiority on two out of three tests of fine motor speed, coordination and strength. In addition, borderline impairments in motor control were seen on the motor aspect of the VMI, recently administered by the school district. These findings are suggestive of a mild relative motor dysfunction in the right hand.

SHERMAN, ADAM
11/01

On the basis of parental report on the ABAS, Adam has mild impairments in personal care, independence and responsibility and severe impairments in the development of social skills. Borderline impairments reported in Adam's communication skills are more reflective of his poor social and pragmatic language skills than of deficits in basic language acquisition.

Mr. Sherman's and Ms. Fuhrman's responses on a parental report inventory (the PIC) are consistent problems related to social skills and peer relationships. Children with similar profiles are likely to experience social isolation and may have difficulty with the regulation of emotions. They may have episodes where their behavior becomes disorganized and may at times experience poor reality testing. In most cases, problems are evident from an early age and may be related to an underlying physiological or genetic disorder.

Adam's responses on a parallel self-report inventory (the PIY) indicate that he is relatively oblivious to his problems. Adam reported that he is a "natural leader" and that he has good relationships with other youngsters. His responses to projective story telling cards suggest poor ability to read emotions and to navigate interpersonal situations. Although his stories indicate that Adam does not seem to expect to be rescued by others, he appears to feel a strong sense of responsibility for helping parental characters that are experiencing distress.

In conclusion, Adam's testing results suggest the presence of a number of mild to moderate deficits in visual processing speed, visual-spatial and visual-constructional skills, social judgement and commonsense. Moderate to severe impairments were seen in verbal and nonverbal abstract and conceptual reasoning and overall cognitive flexibility. Despite average ability to attend to a single stimulus, Adam's ability to shift his attention flexibly between competing stimuli is mildly impaired. Adam requires more time than is typical to consolidate new memories and demonstrates severe deficits in his ability to organize complex, novel visual information for effective storage and retrieval. Inconsistent functioning was seen on tests of fine motor speed, coordination and strength that suggest a mild relative motor dysfunction in the right hand.

Borderline impairments in visual-motor integration, motor control and writing composition were seen in a recent school evaluation. In addition, the school district evaluation documented relative weaknesses in reading comprehension in comparison to reading decoding skills, as well as between math computation as opposed to math reasoning skills.

On the basis of parental report, Adam suffers from mild impairments in the development of personal care, independence and responsibility and severe impairments in social skills. In addition, despite considerable interest in others, Adam has a history of significant impairments in social and emotional interaction. Clinical data and observation suggest that Adam has little understanding of the nature of his social and neurocognitive difficulties.

In light of Adam's strong interest in human relationships and the pattern of his current strengths and deficits, at present his problems seem best described as falling within the spectrum of a neurologically based nonverbal learning disability.

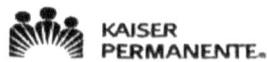 

Case Documents (1300)

CONFIDENTIAL REPORT

Autism Spectrum Disorders Center
Serving Kaiser Permanente families and children with Autism Spectrum Disorders

175 Bernal Road, Suite 230 ♦ San Jose, CA 95119 ♦ Phone (408)362-4350 ♦ Fax (408)362-4355

Autism Spectrum Disorders Center
MULTIDISCIPLINARY EVALUATION SUMMARY

Patient:	Adam Sherman
Kaiser MR #:	10708934
Date of Consultation:	8-4-06
DOB:	November 26, 1991
Age:	14 Years 3 Months
Parents Names:	Spencer Sherman and Janice Fuhrman

EVALUATION PARTICIPANTS
Patient
Parents
Louise Kindell, Psy.D., Psychology Assistant
Pilar Bernal, M.D., Child and Adolescent Psychiatrist

EVALUATION PROCEDURES
Review of Patient Records
Clinical interview with Parent and Child
Completed ASD Parents Orientation Packet
Direct Behavioral and Developmental Observation
Developmental History Questionnaire
Ages & Stages Questionnaire
DBC: Developmental Behavioral Checklist
Achenbach Child Behavior Checklist (Parents, Teacher)
ADOS-G: Autism Diagnostic Observation Schedule, Generic

REFERRAL & CHIEF CONCERNS
Adam was referred to the Autism Spectrum Disorders Center at Kaiser Permanente Santa Teresa Medical Center by Kathy Ray, L.C.S.W from Kaiser Walnut Creek for clarification of diagnosis. His parents report that he has undergone previous evaluations which rendered diagnoses of Aspergers and non-verbal learning disorder. His parents are seeking diagnostic clarification and appropriate treatment recommendations/planning.

BACKGROUND INFORMATION AND CURRENT HISTORY – Obtained from parent interview, parent completed questionnaire and review of reports from past evaluations.

Origin of Concerns:
Adam's parents were first concerned about him when he was approximately three-and-a-half years old. At this time he would not join other children on the playground; he avoided physical activities and sat alone. Much of his play was non-functional and repetitive in nature.

Social Information:
Adam lives with his parents and a younger brother in Lafayette, CA. English is the only language spoken in the home.

Birth and Medical History:

Prenatal Information:	There were no prenatal complications or exposures to toxins.
Birth Information:	Born two weeks early without complications by vaginal delivery.
Hospitalizations:	When tonsils removed; unremarkable
Surgeries:	Tonsils removed
Significant Illnesses or Injuries	Many ear infections. Has scoliosis
Seizures:	None
Medical Studies:	Fragile X testing normal Karyotype negative (at UCSF)
Vision:	No parental concerns
Hearing:	No parental concerns
Medications:	None
Allergies:	No known allergies
Sleep:	No concerns
Eating:	When he was younger would only eat white foods. No current concerns
Elimination	No concerns
Current Health	Healthy.

Family History:
Remarkable for depression, endocrine problems, some family members with "aloof" and "eccentric" behaviors, developmental delays and thyroid problems.

Mental Health History:
In the third grade he began receiving group services at Kaiser. Adam has been receiving counseling services through Kaiser Walnut Creek Psychiatry on a monthly basis for the past year.

Past Behavioral and Developmental Assessments:
Reports from the following previous evaluations were reviewed as part of this assessment:
- Psychoeducational Assessment Report, Layfayette School District (dated 1/26/05)
- Educational Evaluation Report, Layfayette School District (dated 1/05)
- Assessment Summary (dated 1/02)
- Assessment Report by Sarah Hall, Ph.D. (dated 11/01)
- Early Childhood Clinic Summary Report (dated 9/17/97)

Educational and Therapeutic Services:
Adam currently attends mainstream 8th grade at Stanley Elementary School in the Lafayette School District. Adam received speech and language services from Kindergarten through the 5th grade for language pragmatics. Recently he attended a social skills group. His school has recently discontinued his Individualized Education Plan.

Early Developmental History:
Adam walked independently at 14 months. Other motor milestones were slightly delayed and he was a "placid" baby. He was toilet trained on time. Adam said his first words at approximately 12 months and combined words into two to three word phrases at 19 months. Although his parents do not recall when sentences emerged, they did not express any concern about language acquisition delays. He continues to display language pragmatic difficulties. There is no history of language regression.

Language Abilities:
Currently Adam speaks in sentences with good vocabulary and grammar. He uses a words in a formal manner and is described as pedantic. As a youngster, Adam did not ask many "why" questions. He repeated phrases and lines from movies, but out of context. For example, when he opened the door he exclaimed, "Happy Birthday Youngsters!" There is no history of immediate echolalia, but he occasionally whispers to himself. He also likes to recite phrases from TV and books (i.e., Harry Potter).

In conversation, Adam tends to "talk at" others rather than engaging in reciprocal conversation. Even with specific training in this area, Adam continues to have difficulties. He can engage in conversations best when he is discussing his favorite topics and can have other conversations if others keep asking him questions.

His gestures are limited to a few such as pointing, waving goodbye, moving his hand to beckon, nodding and shaking his head. He does not use descriptive gestures. Adam has difficulty with multi-step directions, but his parents have not been particularly concerned with his receptive language. Sometimes Adam will interpret what others say in a literal way and has difficulty understanding jokes, euphuisms and idioms.

Reciprocal and Social Interactions:
His eye contact is poor with those he doesn't know but better with his parents. When Adam was younger he did not approach other children. When he was with other children he engaged in mostly parallel play. Historically and currently, Adam tends to monopolize play with his peers and insist that others follow his interests or take a more passive role. Generally, he enjoys being with children younger than him.

When Adam was younger he did not spontaneously join in and try to copy the actions in social games such as peek-a-boo and patty-cake. He enjoyed having a book read to him
He likes it when his parents read a book to him. Adam has always shown his excitement/interests with his parents by showing and/or talking about them.

Currently, Adam talks at length about other peers at school, but does not have close friendships. He tends to miss social cues and does not seem to understand the complexities of social dynamics. Adam has one friend who calls on an infrequent, but regular basis (this friend has same interests).

Adam has a history of being bullied in the 6th, 7th, and 8th grade. In middle school he formed an environmental club called the "Earth Club" and talks about being popular and wanting to gain even more popularity. Additionally, his parents note he does things "for attention" (ie., break dancing and singing in front of people at school). Currently, Adam is forming a "secret society" for his first year of high school in an attempt to meet popular teens. He talks about this club with his parents and is planning on telling the principle.

Play/ Interests, Routines and Behaviors:
Adam enjoys computes, reading, his Earth Club, and also plays basketball. He is overly preoccupied with forming his new club. Growing up, Adam's interests and play consisted mostly of re-enacting scenes from videotapes. He did not engage in other forms of pretend play.

Adam is not particularly rigid about his routines such as his diet, schedule, placement of objects, things he says and the clothes he wears. He does not however liked to be told at the "last minute" that plans are changing or he is expected to go out.

Adam does not engage in any sensory preoccupations such as looking out of the corner of his eyes, sniffing or licking objects and inappropriately feeling things. He has some tactile sensitivities and enjoys having a blanket wrapped around his shoulders. When he was younger; the clothing tags bothered him. He is also bothered by certain noises such as dogs barking and covers his ears when he hears such noises.

Adam does not flap his hands or exhibit any other unusual movements and did not have any of these behaviors when he was younger. He exhibits some motor tics (began in first grade and was variable throughout the ensuing years) that are very subtle (mild head nodding) and not very noticeable to others.

Adam was described as a very sweet and cooperative child. He apparently had difficulty with transitions when he was younger, but was generally a happy child. He parents deny any history of temper tantrums. Recently when he is angry Adam describes him self feeling very upset, however he controls his behaviors and does not lash out.

EVALUATION PROCEDURES

Autism Diagnostic Observation Schedule (ADOS):
Children with autism spectrum disorders share some critical developmental and behavioral characteristics. In particular they have deficiencies in communication, socialization and rigid adherence to routines. These domains were investigated via interview and observation.

The observation was performed using the Autism Diagnostic Observation Schedule (ADOS). The ADOS, developed by Catherine Lord Ph.D. et. al., is a semi-structured, standardized assessment of communication, social interaction, and play or imaginative use of materials for individuals who have been referred because of possible autism or other pervasive developmental disorders. Administration consists of a series of planned social occasions or "presses" in which a behavior of a particular type is likely to occur. Across the session the examiner presents numerous opportunities for the individual being assessed to exhibit behaviors of interest in the diagnosis process.

15 25 1 70

Module 4 was selected as Adam is verbally fluent and old enough to have been exposed to more mature themes.

Language and Communication
Adam uses sentences in a largely correct fashion. He has a noticeably mechanical way of speaking with little variation in his pitch and tone. Additionally, his speech is at times abnormal in volume. He demonstrates no immediate echolalia. He tends to use his words and phrases in a particularly formal manner.

Adam does well spontaneously offing information about his own thoughts, feelings and experiences. He did not ask any information of this examiner upon administration of the ADOS. Adam reported a specific nonroutine event in a reasonable manner and was able to sustain a flowing conversation. His gestures were conventional and instrumental in nature, but Adam did not use descriptive gestures. He had some emphatic or emotional gestures, but they were limited in frequency.

Reciprocal Social Interaction
Adam had fairly appropriate gaze with subtle changes meshed with other communication. His facial expressions were somewhat limited and he linked his vocalizations with socially appropriate changes in gesture, gaze and facial expression. He seemed to have little expressed pleasure in interaction and showed more pleasure from his own actions and part of the conversation. He had some description of his own emotions and demonstrated understanding of the experience of another (i.e., friend was upset over Earth Club interaction).

Adam demonstrated some insight into several typical social relationships, but not necessarily his own role. Adam discussed his responsibility in various contexts. He had some slightly unusual quality of social overtures and such overtures were restricted to his own interests. The quality of social response was somewhat limited and socially awkward, and the frequency of reciprocal social communication was slightly limited. The overall quality of rapport was comfortable, but not sustained as Adam's behavior was at times awkward or stilted.

Imagination
Adam used several different spontaneous, inventive, creative activities or comments in conversation.

Stereotyped Behaviors and Restricted Interests
He demonstrated no unusual sensory interest in play material/person, no hand/finger or other complex mannerisms and no self-injurious behaviors. Adam did have unusual patterns of interest (i.e., environmentalism and being popular) that at times interfered with social communication. He had no obvious compulsions or rituals.

Other Abnormal Behaviors
Adam sat still and had no disruptive behavior. He was mildly anxious at times, especially in response to social presses.

Overall ADOS Impressions

Adam's scores on the ADOS algorithm exceeded the threshold score for "autism spectrum range," on the Communication domain and exceeded the threshold score for "autism range" and Reciprocal Social Interaction domains. Their combined score exceeded the threshold score for "autism range." Although no threshold scores are available for the Imagination/Creativity domain, he displayed difficulties in this area. His score on the domain of Stereotyped Behaviors and Restricted Interests, also without any available threshold, suggests some difficulties. Overall, the results of the ADOS indicate that Adam displays behaviors that are seen in children with an autism spectrum disorder.

Adaptive Assessment:

Adaptive Behavior Assessment System, 2nd Ed. (ABAS-II)
The ABAS-II measures the functional skills of individuals from birth to adulthood necessary for daily living, focusing on what they do without help from others and whether they do them when needed. Adaptive behavior scores measure whether an individual performs the correct behavior or skill when it is needed, which is very different from just saying that someone knows how to perform a behavior. These scales, therefore, assess what a person actually does as opposed to what he or she is capable of doing. The ABAS-II covers adaptive behaviors in three different domains: Conceptual (communication and academic skills), Social (interpersonal and social competence skills), and Practical (independent living and daily living skills). It also provides a General Adaptive Composite (GAC) score that summarizes the individual's performance across all of these domains.

Interpretation: The standard scores reported have a mean of 100 and a standard deviation (SD) of 15, thus allowing direct comparisons to "IQ"-type standard scores on common intelligence tests. Standard scores within one SD encompass 90-110 and include about 68% of individuals in a given age and scores two SDs (80-120) include 82%. Scores below 70 suggest significant deficits on that domain. The Band of Error scores are those that are 90% to contain the individual's true score.

Domain	Standard Scores	Band of Error 90% CI	90%-ile Rank	Adaptive Level
GAC	72	85-91	21%	Below Average
Conceptual	26	88-96	30%	Average
Social	13	83-93	21%	Below Average
Practical	31	83-93	21%	Below Average

Adam displays deficits in his adaptive behaviors across some assessed domains. His lowest rated abilities were in the subdomains of:
- Community Use (i.e., navigating and functioning in the outside world)
- Home Living (i.e., doing chores and cleaning up after himself)
- Social (i.e., having friends and interacting appropriately with other people).

Adam was reported to have a relatively higher level of abilities in his ability to participate in health and safety, self-care and self-direction skills.

SubDomain	Raw Score	Scaled Score	Age Equivalency Years:months
Conceptual -Communication	63	9	9:0-9:3
Conceptual – Functional Academics	58	7	10-10:3
Conceptual – Self-Direction	62	10	14:0-14:11

Social –Leisure	52	8	8:4-8:7
Social –Social	51	6	<5:0
Practical –Community Use	42	7	9:8-9:11
Practical –Home Living	48	3	8:4-8:7
Practical –Health & Safety	61	11	15:0-15:11
Practical –Self-Care	70	10	>12:11

His ratings of adaptive behavior indicate that, despite a lack of significant cognitive impairments, his daily functioning at the level of a younger child in many areas. Such a pattern is typical of children with high-functioning autistic spectrum disorders. His scores indicate that communication, behavioral, and social skill areas of development should be targeted for development at both home and school.

IMPRESSIONS

Evaluation Summary

Adam is a 14-year-old healthy male who presents with difficulties in several areas of functioning, despite his good cognitive abilities. Socialization and the ability to initiate and sustain peer relationships pose a challenge for Adam. A lack of social reciprocity, missing social cues and a limited understanding regarding the rules that govern socialization contribute to difficulties in this area. Although Adam has no significant speech delays, he struggles with social pragmatics and having a to-and-fro conversation on different topics. Adam also displays encompassing restricted ranges of interests (i.e., environmentalism). Despite these challenges, Adam has many strengths. He is described as a loving and good-natured individual with many ideas who is loved by his family a great deal. The following treatment recommendations will likely further Adam's development (please see below). At this time, a diagnosis of Aspergers best explains Adam's presenting problems.

DSM-IV Diagnostic Criteria for Autism

Marked	None	Diagnostic Category
X		Impairment in the use of multiple nonverbal behaviors such as eye-to-eye gaze, facial expression, body postures, and gestures to regulate social interactions.
X		Failure to develop peer relationships appropriate to developmental level.
	X	Lack of spontaneous seeking to share enjoyment, interests, or achievements with other people (e.g., by a lack of showing, bringing, or pointing out objects of interest).
X		Lack of social or emotional reciprocity.

Marked	None	Diagnostic Category
	X	Delay in, or total lack of, the development of spoken language (not accompanied by an attempt to compensate through alternative modes of communication such as gesture or mime)
X		In individuals with adequate speech, marked impairment in the ability to initiate or sustain a conversation with others.
	X	Stereotyped and repetitive use of language or idiosyncratic language.
	X	Lack of varied, spontaneous make-believe play or social imitative play appropriate to developmental level.

Marked	None	Diagnostic Category
X		Encompassing preoccupation with one or more stereotyped and restricted patterns of interest that is abnormal either in intensity or focus.

CHAPTER 4
ON THE SURFACE

In medias res
Stand your ground. Show them no quarter. Cowardice will not be tolerated. Those were the thoughts that resonated in my mind partway into my first year of high school, for that was the time when I was seeing much of my community for what it truly was: deceitful and ignorant. Before descending into its depths, however, there is still the surface I have barely scratched that I must describe first.

Flashback: three years earlier
The year after my dispute with K.P., my parents moved us for the fifth and final time to a small dot of a town called Lafayette, situated on the eastern end of the San Francisco Bay Area. On the surface, it was a beautiful place to live. Our house was a gray, three-story quasi-pyramid-shaped building, set against a sloping hill with a view of the town and valley below it. It felt as if we were on the edge of nature and society: the cars, the people and the other houses in front, and in back a green, endless forest, sweeping up the mountain and stretching through bigger hills and valleys and around a local reservoir, picturesque to all who visited the area. To my family, it was paradise, but to me it was a prison, for despite recent events with my first crush, I still considered the town we previously lived in to be my home and was not forgiving toward my father for taking his third new job in the last nine years of my life and uprooting our lives once again. Caring, calm, and patient as ever, my father promised me that this move was permanent, at least while I was still in school, and that being here, in a small town connected to the bigger

cityscape beyond the hills in San Francisco, would open up more educational opportunities. My mother also believed that it would expose my brother and me to a wider world that we had yet to live in, and that staying in a small town like Napa would prevent that from taking place. Still skeptical of the new situation, as I had been previously with our other moves, I reluctantly accepted this.

My first difficulty, while nascent at first, came when I entered middle school and quickly realized that I had walked into a society where most of my classmates had a more stationary life and had known each other since they were toddlers. They all had their predetermined social groups and were interested in hobbies, pop culture, and music I had never heard of. In some ways, it felt like they had their own language, one that only they understood and a newcomer like me did not, which made it all sound like noise and increased my social anxiety and subsequent introversion. I was instantly labeled an outsider, as I struggled to understand the kind of world they were living in. My teachers were the first ones I began to trust, as most of them were kind and considerate and gave me the perfect distraction from my social difficulties: homework and projects. Many people at my age considered an interest in schoolwork to be nothing short of insanity, as we were still kids who should have wanted nothing more than to enjoy our lives.

While I remained a diligent student throughout middle school, my classmates' viewpoint eventually spurred me on to make a few friends, and by the end of my first year, I was part of a *Three Musketeers* group consisting of me, Z.M., and S.S., who quickly proved their loyalty by spending most days of the week with me in and out of school, and even went as far as to protect me from a school bully who liked going after the new, insecure kids (*in truth, however, I could have defended myself, courtesy of four years of martial arts experience*). Z.M. was a short, scrawny boy with a mess of curly brown hair and loose-hanging clothes, usually oversized shorts and T-shirts, though with the occasional flannel and carpenter jeans. He had a face with straight features that looked permanently quizzical and had a curious nature, though he was also somewhat introverted like me. S.S. was the exact opposite; he was taller and sturdier with short, sandy-blond hair, and he mostly wore shorts and shirts that hugged his frame, where even at his young age, he looked like he had the body of a surfer. His face was lightly freckled and had more finely carved features with an air of cool confidence that further added credibility to his surfer look. Thanks to them, the rest of middle school became easier, and even girls began to show an interest in me by approaching me to talk. Before long, the more popular kids took notice and invited me to be a part of their group as well. I also got to know students from other walks of life. In short, I began to convince myself that I had the ability to make friends and establish good relationships with people of all backgrounds, social statuses, and cliques, and this further fed my growing belief that I was a friend to all in my social environment.

An idea started it all. A childhood cartoon gave me the idea, and I was quick to make it a reality with my parents' help. As a newly minted thirteen-year-old, I believed I had stepped into a gold mine, the gold in question being the many aluminum cans, plastic and glass bottles found in my house, my neighborhood, and my school. Collecting these and turning them over to a recycling plant put money into my hands and made for a cleaner school and environment. In turn, I learned the value of community service, as well as operating a rudimentary business with my friends, evenly distributing their hard-earned money and drawing admiration and support from the school staff (*I later discovered that my principal, while knowing it was against the rules for a student to make a profit on school grounds, let it slide when he saw the good I was doing for the school and how much my heart was devoted to it*). What followed was the founding of a club where the proceeds went to the school, a routine to clean up the grounds after hours and eventually, being awarded the second highest honor at graduation for my "selfless service to the school," as told by the vice principal.

Mixed in with all of that, however, was a gradual realization that not everyone supported my actions; some did not care, and others considered it weird and against the norms of their community. There were isolated incidents at first, from an occasional insult to someone knocking over our collection cart. For a "normal," confident kid like me with a support system, it was easy for me to play these off, and I often added new ideas to expand awareness of my recycling and community service in order to foment support and outweigh opposition. I still had everything I wanted and needed out of life, my sense of hard work was growing, my friendships were far stronger than my fears of being confronted by the more antagonistic people in school, and near the end of my time in middle school, I had better relationships with the girls in my school and the growing confidence to get to know them on a more personal level.

The beginning of high school started with a sense of calm and optimism that had never before burned so brightly within me. I was moving up with the same people I had gotten to know for the last three years, I felt more accepted than in the beginning, and I had already made a positive name for myself in my community. Or so I thought. One visit to the Santa Clara medical clinic, and the ride home changed all of that. The events that followed revealed a truth that I had been so blind to, and made it all the more difficult to accept with the impervious wall of denial that followed me home.

CHAPTER 5
BLOODY KNUCKLES AND BOLD-FACED LIES

Present day
Flowing like water, tasting like vinegar, running all over my fist like lava from a volcano as I stood over the man lying flat on his back. The reality was nothing like that, but in my mind's eye, in my heart, I felt like it was. Freshman year of high school started off well, as I still had my core friends, even though one of them (S.S.) went to another school and the other one (Z.M.) was, thankfully, starting this new journey with me. I still believed that my relationships with other people crossed every social boundary, every grade, and every interest, and with the success of middle school, this would be a step toward my true potential. Any thought of my being socially inept and developmentally disabled was tucked away in a forgotten corner of my mind, as the "wall" was proving capable of keeping such thoughts at bay and allowing me to live my life. My parents had heeded my warning and were letting me decide what I wanted to do with my life, with certain conditions attached, such as having a sport to keep me busy and healthy and finding jobs outside of school. Within the first month of school I was doing well in most of my classes, making friends with the upperclassmen, joining the cross-country team, and deciding to run for freshman class vice president.

At that moment I was certain that I had the backing of my class, as I had seemingly gained their friendship, trust, and respect. I believed that the perfect high school experience was already coming together and that I would be an example of a normal kid reaching his fullest potential.

That illusion cracked like a rock thrown into a mirror, shattering the glass into fine pieces. This first event was, for me, the beginning of my descent into the dark and murky abyss that became my reality of high school. After giving what I thought was a rousing speech to my freshman class, I went through the rest of the day with a confidence that went as high as the beautiful, sunny sky above the campus. I reflected on what went into my campaign: numerous posters with a Clint Eastwood *Dirty Harry* theme, a massive banner that spanned half of the north wing of the school, numerous flyers passed out and lying across the benches for people to read, and even a fun little rap music video I made, thinking that adding light-heartedness and going off of a suggestion to "put myself out there" would help even more. Everyone knew my name and face, and I was so proud of myself, thinking that I was about to be a student body representative who did right by his friends and classmates and made our experiences better for everyone.

The bell rang at the end of my final class and the puddle of mud was the first thing I saw as I crossed the courtyard toward the parking lot. However, the puddle was not its usual brown color; for some reason, it looked blue. Curious, I approached the puddle, and to my shock, I saw my face peering out of the muck. The numerous pixelated inkblots that made up my face, giving the same Clint Eastwood look to go with the theme, stared back at me, as if desperately trying not to sink into dirty oblivion. I reached down to pick up what was once a proud-looking flyer and quickly realized it was part of a stack of them that had been tossed into the mud, some of them looking like they had shoe prints on them as if they had been stomped deeper and deeper into the wet dirt. I knew immediately that something was wrong. My heart sank into the pit of my stomach as I raced back to the north wing of the school, and a scene of devastation hit me like a ton of bricks: my flyers ripped and shredded and tossed all over the quad, my posters defaced and marked with obscenities, and my precious banner nowhere to be found. The shock anchored me where I was for some time, for as terrible as this was to look at, I found I could not tear my eyes away. Eventually, I managed to stagger back toward the parking lot to get picked up and then went home to tell my parents what had happened. They promptly reported the incident to the school, though in the back of my mind, the damage was already done. I had a good idea of why this was done and what was coming next.

A penchant for my worst fears coming true began in earnest, starting when suddenly I was being mocked by the very people I thought were my friends for my somewhat flamboyant music video, with direct insults and obscenities included in their taunts. What followed was an election where my opponent won by a landslide and culminated in a visit to the principal with my parents, who informed us that not only did I barely get any votes (*thirty-seven to be exact*) but that the targeted vandalism of my campaign was unlike anything the school had ever experienced, certainly nothing he nor the leadership class had ever encountered. Despite this admission, he went on to say that although this was a serious matter, he did not believe that they could launch a proper investigation and apologized for my ordeal. This response puzzled me, for not only was this a unique event in the school's history, but there were also security cameras all around the school, a proctor who patrolled the hallways, and a so-called "honor code" in place to create a safer and more inclusive environment. My mother would go on to say that he was a weak and cowardly man for not looking into the matter (*in contrast to his strong, tall stature and imposing personality; he would later become superintendent for the district*).

As we left the main office I noticed something etched into the wall on the side of the entrance to the building. It was artwork shaped like a tree, only this tree did not contain leaves, but tags with the names of "booster" parents and other donors to the school. The majority of those names, particularly the last names, were ones I immediately recognized as those belonging to the people who had turned on me. It then dawned on me why the principal was so quick to shoot down any investigation into the personal attack on my character. I learned two things that day: the school was in the pocket of wealthy donors and would prioritize them over my safety without a second thought, and this would be the catalyst that would propel me to develop into someone who would fight to hold people and institutions like my school responsible for their actions or lack thereof.

The student body began to thoroughly play its part in the continued disruption of my everyday life. It was as if an infectious disease of hate mixed with ignorance to my different social personality had corrupted those within my class and those of the lower grades as my four years of high school slowly ground on, and the true extent of that disease became known with every passing day. In my first year, shortly after the disastrous student leadership elections, I was walking through the halls near where my banner was stolen when some people from the in crowd came up to me. In middle school I had developed a talent for impromptu singing on request and was consistently told that I had a good singing voice. They asked me if they could relive those days again and, with my wall of denial in place and hoping that this would bring back some normalcy, I obliged.

I had barely begun the first chorus of my song when one particular person, G.C., interrupted me in a wild fashion. He was a shrimp of a person, hardly more than two-thirds my height (*six foot two inches*), yet he had a reputation for refusing to be intimidated by anyone. On this day, G.C. was dressed in slightly torn denim jeans and a white hoodie that could be zipped up over his head and cover him like someone in a full-body spandex outfit. That was the first thing I noticed before he blindly launched himself at me, grabbed my arm, and attempted to pull me to the ground. His other hand reached up as if to grab the back of my head and wipe the ground with my face. He never got the chance, for in a split second I threw a boxing punch known as a right-across and hit him square in the middle of his forehead, to which he crumpled to the ground instantly. For a split second I stood there, frozen in shock at what I had done, violent images flashing in my mind's eye, which was immediately followed by strong feelings of guilt and remorse, at which I then promptly bolted from the scene without turning back to witness the shock and amazement on the faces of those who, just moments ago, were listening to the cover of their favorite song. As I paced the hallways, praying for the lunch break to be over so I could quickly duck into my next class, the concept of Sir Isaac Newton's third law of motion jumped into my head, that "for every action there is an equal and opposite reaction," and I had to prepare for the potential consequences of what my actions had caused. However, discipline from the school never came; instead, I would soon discover that I had poked the beast in the eye, something worse than any punishment the school could have given me, and that the repercussion would prove to be one I would never have been able to anticipate or prepare for.

CHAPTER 6
ESCALATION AT ITS FINEST

Physical confrontation was inevitable. That much was certain, and the certainty presented itself when I was ambushed in the locker room later that day by G.C. and several of his friends. I managed to hold my own, however, and after much shoving around the lockers, they gave up, especially when the sound of our physical education teacher arriving carried through the nearby hall. Naively, I believed the worst was over, as not even the boys with the physique of a sports star had been able to put me in my place, so it appeared that those confrontations were already in the rear-view mirror.

One day, I was enjoying my lunch in the quad when a tall senior boy approached me. He had on black shoes that were thoroughly worn, jeans frayed at the seams, and a black hoodie pulled over a baseball cap from which a tangle of long, brown hair flowed down his shoulders on either side of his rough, severely unshaven face. He was eighteen years old, like many of the seniors in my high school, but he looked ten years older. There was something in his eyes that seethed, yet they also appeared to be strangely out of focus. He did not seem to be fixated on hate, more of a sense of intimidation. Out of the corner of my eye I saw my fellow freshman classmates watching us, talking excitedly, holding their food like popcorn at the movies, some of them unable to hide their glee at what was unfolding in front of them.

In many ways, it was more terrifying than what went down in the locker room weeks before. The bloodcurdling scream that jumped from his lips was sudden and deafening. Compared with the average person, my five senses were, and still are, ultra-sensitive, especially my hearing, so it came as no surprise that I jumped several feet back and into the air. He then began yelling nonsense and taking wild swipes at me, his eyes crazed and unfocused, spittle oozing from the sides of his mouth like a rabid dog. The swipes kept coming, and people continued to watch and did nothing as the scene unfolded in front of them. Finally, after about a minute (which felt like an hour) another senior came up and calmed him down, escorting him away while talking slowly and calmly to him, leaving me to absorb the shock of what had happened and the continuous stares from the crowd. By the end of the school day, I decided to do some investigating, and through my research I discovered that the senior boy, A.M., was part of "Learning Skills," a class designed for people who were struggling academically due to mental challenges. While it was not a class for the truly mentally disabled (*Down syndrome, low-functioning autism, etc.*) it nonetheless catered to those who have learning and social disorders, and A.M. was a part of that class. I then flashed back to the scene in the quad where I saw a number of the freshman boys, people whom I thought were my friends, watching with wicked smiles and anticipation akin to that of gladiator combat in the Roman Colosseum. With a jolt, I realized that they had sent him after me like a trained pit bull, manipulating him into scaring me half to death and attacking me the way they could not without getting caught. All those few years since moving to Lafayette where I thought I had made a stable and trusting web of friends and acquaintances were beginning to unravel in earnest.

From that point on, the foundations of my life in school and in the community began to crumble. During a routine cross-country practice, I found myself running alone near the end of the course my coaches had set for us. It was a nice, quiet stretch of woodland that ran next to the school, and I was only a quarter mile away from finishing. Upon reaching the turn that led to the street that would take me back to the field for cool-down stretching, a half dozen boys dressed in black jumped out of the trees, the biggest of them preparing to rush me with a large, wooden baseball bat. I recognized him as P.F-S., a stout, overweight boy with a wild tangle of dirty-brown hair whom I had gone to middle school with. He had a massive temper and frequent troubles with both the school and the law, and even though he went to another school, he appeared to be leading this group from my school in an attack on me. In his eyes, I saw the lust for power and control burning alongside the rage; P.F-S. was thoroughly enjoying this moment, ready to bring down the bat on top of my head with all of the strength he could muster from his broad arms and shoulders. He would have definitely followed through, if not for the poor choice of location. While I was not yet back at the field, there was a clearing that one could view the field from, and the entire junior varsity football team was practicing, with a few players just noticing what was happening two hundred yards away. The boys backed off, disappearing back into the woods as quickly as they had appeared like a swarm of insects, and I subsequently made a dash for the safety of the stadium and my fellow runners.

The next confrontation happened during my sophomore year at the homecoming dance. After unsuccessfully trying to dance with several girls, five in-crowd guys surrounded me and then began "freaking" me, grinding up against me the way they always did with the other girls on the dance floor. While in hindsight I realized they were trying to embarrass me and acting like complete fools, at that moment I thought it was another attack, and I did not hesitate to use a double elbow strike to knock two of them down and hit the others in their collarbones while I ran for the exit. While no further physical confrontations happened that night, the damage was done; they had intimidated me enough that I did not plan to go to another school dance again.

The threat of physical violence melted away after that encounter but evolved into bigger and far more sinister forms as time went on. It appeared that there was almost no low that many of my classmates would not sink to if it meant hurting me any way they could, and they continuously succeeded at not getting caught by the school or the authorities. Despite being the target, I saw myself taking note of how they went about their methods of intimidation, confrontation, and fabrication of stories about me. It always seemed to start with those who had the highest social standing, and from there it would trickle down into the other social circles of the school, and in some cases, reach the ears of those in other schools and communities. As much as I tried to convince myself that I could overcome any challenge I came up against, this constantly evolving situation found ways to affect me in the worst, most unexpected ways, and this series of misfortunes and deliberately staged events would continue in manners that would far exceed any kind of comprehension I had at the time.

CHAPTER 7
EMPIRES FALL

The web had disintegrated, the strands coming apart and falling away as they were cut by the people I had spent several years believing to be my friends, the dream of being a friend to all dissolving and tearing apart, my glass-completely-full attitude beginning to spill at a considerable rate. Despite the empire that I thought had been my social life being overrun by the barbaric acts of my peers, I took some comfort knowing that not all was lost, for I still had a core group of friends who had stood by me for years, in addition to a dear friend from another school who was always there for me and was always willing to help me through the roughest periods of my life. In addition to the support of my teachers and the unconditional love of my family, I still felt that I could ride out the storm surrounding me at school.

It all started with an impulse. Despite having a best friend like Z.M. by my side, I was not his best friend, for he had a best friend, M.B., whom he had known for much longer than me. M.B. was a year older than us and unassuming, usually dressed in loose-fitting jeans and a dark sweatshirt, his short, sandy-colored hair constantly covered by a baseball cap, and his facial features giving a rather blank and almost sullen look. Despite his appearance I was not bothered by it, nor his friendship with Z.M., as he was just as much a part of our core circle of friends, from his loyalty to his common interests in pop culture and generally being silly with each other. One other thing we also had in common was that we were not the most developmentally accomplished of people either. In one of his few moments of vulnerability, I discovered that, like me, Z.M. also had a hard time understanding certain people on a social level, quite possibly being autistic as well, and the other friends we had in our group were considered a part of the aforementioned "Learning Skills" class, ranging from Tourette's syndrome to general social anxiety, which gave me comfort knowing that we still had each other despite our shared hardships. That alone was enough for me to appreciate what I still had in my life as opposed to what I had lost. So how could I possibly have thought with this kind of support that anything could go wrong?

During my first year of high school it was all about the mania surrounding the Star Wars prequel trilogy, and another friend of mine, A.T. a tall, skinny boy with short curly black hair and glasses dressed in khaki shorts and an orange T-shirt, had shown me a video of two ordinary guys who, through the use of special effects, created an epic lightsaber battle. We decided to do a similar lightsaber battle in the quad during lunch, as we had already seen many other people acting out Star Wars battles in anticipation of the final film in the trilogy. In that moment, we had fun acting out the battle, rolling around on the grass, miming lightsabers in our hands, and using martial arts techniques to make it look choreographed and professional. However, as I would quickly discover, not only did we make complete fools of ourselves in front of our class, but M.B. also witnessed our act and became upset and offended, which resulted in an angry voicemail from him after school telling me that we were finished and that he never wanted to speak or associate with me ever again.

My reaction was swift. My movements became slow and heavy as if I were dragging weights from my back, my mind quickly immobilized by shock, the deep dark dread in the back of my mind beginning to filter out into the other corners of my head like hot tar in the street. This was the last thing in the world I had expected to happen, and I immediately went into damage control, wanting to make things right as soon as possible. A few days later I approached him and apologized for my actions, telling him I had never meant to offend anyone and that I would stop doing those antics I had displayed in the quad, and vowed to be a better person. M.B. immediately and viciously rejected my apology and went on to openly mock me in front of the entire freshman class, ridiculing me as an attention-seeking loser who had no redeeming qualities whatsoever and vowing to never forgive me for the rest of his life. Throughout his punishing verbal blows, out of the corner of my eyes I saw dozens of people staring at us, listening with rapt attention at every word that came out of his mouth, with a few of the boys looking quite amused at the bullying that was happening to me. Embarrassed and emotionally broken by his outburst and die-hard conviction, I quietly bowed my head and walked away, disappearing into an empty wing of the school. Confusion and depression covered me like a shroud, as I was certain that because of this, I had lost every friend I had, for I was convinced that Z.M. would listen to him and desert me as well. For the most part it was true, as the other two friends in the group stood by him, with one (S.J.) insulting me in a Tourette's syndrome–induced rage and the other (C.C.) outright running away every time he saw me.

Z.M., however, accepted my apology and remained by my side, even cementing my respect and loyalty when, as a birthday present, he helped me get my first job at a movie theater he worked at. I was grateful to him for this generous act and made it known when we were working together, for we both were major fans of cinema and enjoyed the benefits that came with working there. I still sensed, however, that there was something going on with him.

It was as if, despite our renewed closeness and our shared interests, there was a part of him that was not there, and I suspected that it was because of M.B. He had told me, upon presenting me with my new job, that M.B. had long held ultra-sensitive beliefs and was easily offended by anything he perceived to be an insult to him. As a result, M.B. had never forgiven anyone he believed had wronged him, which proved the futility of my previous efforts. Z.M. assured me that he was nothing like that and I did not question him any further, despite how certain I was that his friend was trying to turn him against me. Six months went by, six months of continued school, work, and play, and for a time there was peace in my life, and not even daily hardships at school or the increasingly difficult volume of homework could keep me down. Then a letter showed up at my door.

It was made the old-fashioned way, hand-written in pencil and on a sheet of lined office paper. I immediately recognized the careful and precise scrawl of Z.M. He described how he had taken time to think about us as friends, and that after much consideration, he had come to the conclusion that M.B. may have been right about me, that I had displayed signs of clinging, excessive gratitude, and an overall disregard for his feelings about a great many things (*he did not specify anything about these perceived issues with me*). He went on the say that if he had to choose between our friendship and his life, that he would always choose himself above all else, and ended the letter by telling me to stay away from his younger brother, whom I had begun a mentoring relationship with in order to make him feel comfortable with transitioning to high school.

The force of slamming into a concrete wall hit my psyche; it was as if I had been stunned, frozen in a place between time and space. Here was the friend whom I had known for well over four years, the friend who stood by me in the face of schoolyard bullies, who shared my interests in movies and passion projects, which included being an integral part of my rudimentary recycling business, who disagreed with what everyone else thought of me and helped me advance my aspirations and developments as a person, suddenly turning around and betraying all of my trust, loyalty, and camaraderie with a few strokes of a pencil. What followed was a wave of despair the likes of which I had never known, for the final person who had unconditionally supported me like my own family had left me for social dead, like so many others. My father attempted to comfort me, saying that he had always suspected that Z.M. was a weak-willed person who sold me out under pressure, but all this did was deepen my depression and make me think that if he could see what I could not, then just how many more relationships of mine were just another in a long list of lies, deceit, and betrayals?

CHAPTER 8
DESPAIR AND DESERTED ISLANDS

Events only became worse from then on. My involvement in school activities was faltering: I quit cross-country and track after I injured my hip during a race and my applications to assist in student leadership were repeatedly turned down. But worst of all, my commitment to the environmental club proved futile. Where the previous leaders during my freshman and sophomore year had seen my potential and loyalty to the cause and groomed me to be their successor, the process was hijacked during my junior year when two classmates brought their friends to the meeting to have themselves elected co-presidents of the club in order to look good for their college applications. More than half of their friends who showed up to vote never returned to future meetings. In addition, the passing of my paternal grandfather during that time led to further ridicule when, instead of respecting me and giving me the space to grieve or provide support through it all, many members of the student body used it to further their exploitation of me and my vulnerable state, often in the form of taunts like calling me a sissy or even declaring that I was not a man for being emotional and appearing weak. These open-season-esque attacks and dehumanizing declarations made my grief all the more unbearable.

Nasty rumors continued to circulate around me as well, rumors that I was a closeted gay man because I had light eye color and talked in a high, effeminate voice, which many small-minded individuals associated with gay men. I attempted to show I was straight by showing genuine interest in, and subsequently asking out, a girl, J.H., whom I had liked for years. But the rumors spread by her clique changed direction and took the form of saying that she was a lesbian because she had a masculine affinity for sports and a deep, slightly husky voice. This soon spread around to further belief and ridicule toward me (*She turned out not to be lesbian, but, being part of the in-crowd, made no attempt to defend me or curtail the rumors*). By Valentine's Day, I had sent an anonymous love note, encouraged by a Leadership class activity, to another girl, S.C., a tall, elegant person with long, flowing dirty-blonde hair, tight-fitting designer clothes and finely carved features of an amateur model, whom I also had strong feelings for. But some people deduced that it was me and pressured both of us with insults, taunts, and borderline threats until she cracked and declared that we could only ever be friends.

Rumors like this built on each other to the point where, despite my best efforts, for the first three years of high school I was never able to get a date to any school dance, including my junior prom, as I was shunned by everyone I had asked. My sixteenth birthday was nothing short of disastrous when I impulsively spread the word that I was planning a major celebration, like many of my rich classmates did, only to have my parents refuse. In one of my lowest moments, one I could never be proud of, I lashed out at them and said terrible, hurtful things, not out of genuine hate, but out of fear of being a laughing stock at school, which is precisely what materialized. It became that much worse when, Z.M. joined a short-lived Facebook group dubbed "The Anti-Sherman Club," created by M.B. and dedicated to the opposition and destruction of my name and existence in school and the community. While it was swiftly shut down by the social media platform and group members reprimanded by their parents and the school, the psychological damage was done.

The very worst, however, occurred in my Spanish class while trying to help my partners with a project. For a couple of days we had been struggling to agree on an idea, so I told them I had finally figured out a solution to our dilemma. Before I knew it, they had spread a rumor that I had espoused Adolf Hitler's "Final Solution" to the Jewish people, knowing full well that I was Jewish and German on my mother's side but my family and ancestors had no ties whatsoever to the Nazis. This particular rumor, I believed, was spread to inflict more emotional pain on me and to leave an indelible mark on my psyche and my sense of self-worth. This felt like a lot more than simply the work of insensitive, privileged teenagers; it felt like the work of certain people who enjoyed causing pain and used their status in school to command loyalty and belief in their gossip and lies. They had no way of knowing—but perhaps would not care if they did—that for many years I would carry a massive amount of guilt due because they had instilled the belief that I should be ashamed to be Jewish and German, because that made me a living representation of the worst atrocity ever committed against the Jews by means of Nazi Germany's Holocaust. Even then, my schoolmates would continue to prove to me that there was no such thing as enough punishment for me at their hands.

For the first few years, I had few to no allies in the fight against an increasingly ignorant and apathetic system that was my high school experience. The school administration was unfeeling and bureaucratic; they were more concerned with running the school and paying attention to the entire student body instead of any one person's suffering. It did not help that I was deferred to the school psychologist, who had no authority beyond analyzing me and advising me about how to stand up and ignore the people making my life difficult. Because of the school's indifference to my situation, my parents did not have much power in forcing things to change. There were many nights that all they could do was listen to how horrible my days at school were, how I could not concentrate or comprehend mathematics and hard sciences (chemistry, physics, etc.), how my grades were suffering overall, how many of my teachers treated me like another number on a checklist, and worse, how in every part of the school, people were looking at me like prey. I could tell they were hurting seeing their son in such pain and seeing my grades and interest in school decline, but in all my pain and denial, I did not care much because they were not me and had no comprehension of my pain.

However, while it lasted, and before the apathetic social hierarchy completely took over the school by my senior year, I had temporary relief from my hardships by making connections with the upperclassmen, for they showed more maturity individually than my entire class put together. Those connections gained me a number of friends, which included Elizabeth "Liz" Blee, who aspired to be a therapist (*and still my friend to this day*); a member of the Student Leadership council; and even two successive captains of the boys' varsity basketball team. The basketball players genuinely appreciated my support for their team and them as people instead of just school icons, for one of them came from humble beginnings and had worked hard to prove himself on the court, while the other one was a genuinely good soul struggling to balance expectations for his team and being inclusive to those around him. While I knew that they would graduate well before I did, I also knew that I needed to enjoy and appreciate these connections while I had them, so I never took any moment for granted. But that was also where I made a mistake: I was inclusive, took everything at face value, and saw nothing but the best in people. While to most those were admirable qualities, it also blinded me to the more subversive undertones of some people and the often overzealous perceptions they exhibited, which also included some of the upperclassmen.

In hindsight, I should have known that there would be at least one person who not only kept secrets, but also allowed for bad things to happen at the expense of others. That person was T.M., a tall, blonde, and athletic-looking girl who took part in galvanizing school spirit for sports and other events. She was a year above me, and in the beginning, was someone whom I looked up to and got along with, perhaps because she recognized my kindness toward her and considered us as an example of unifying the underclassmen with the upperclassmen through friendship and school spirit. Shortly after I was hired at the movie theater, I was passing by the community pool and saw her working there as a lifeguard. I stopped by to visit, and we had a great conversation in which she expressed how happy she was that I found such a great place to work, and she invited me to stop by whenever I wanted to check up on her and tell her how my day went. Being someone I trusted, I honored that request and came by two to three days a week whenever I finished work. At first it was pleasant, but then I was blindsided.

I had arrived at the pool after work, and as T.M. was approaching the gate to talk to me while locking up the area, a van pulled up and several women about her age and older jumped out. They ambushed me, backing me against a wall, looks of the deepest, vindictive fury and disgust on their faces. I was scared and confused and wondering where this was coming from and why. They began accusing me of harassment and stalking (*second time in my life I heard that word*), telling me that I was intruding on both a sanctuary for families and for the staff, which included T.M. Completely bewildered and in shock, I stammered to them that I was here to see a friend, that was all I had ever been doing, and that they were way out of line to accuse me of something so horrific. I then turned to T.M. and begged her to back me up and explain that to them. She briefly struggled to respond, then quickly and almost fluidly, gave in and warned me not to come see her anymore, as it was negatively affecting her job and her standing with the staff and community. Shock and a sense of betrayal set in, and I hung my head and took off on my bike heading home, burning with sadness and humiliation at what had just transpired.

After the summer ended, I planned to confront her about what she had done and find out why she would betray me in such a public fashion, only to discover she was no longer attending my school. Later I found out that T.M. had been caught in possession of a large amount of drugs (allegedly cocaine) and had been sent to a disciplinary boarding school in Arizona. The realization set in that despite the initially sweet and angelic image she had cultivated, she had a more subversive, devious side to her that I had been blind to. As a result, she was the wrong kind of person to have in my circle of friends, but I been unable to see what was beneath the surface.

Throughout these unfortunate events, I felt my mental and physical health suffer greatly. The shutting down of most of my relationships in school and the broader community had reached a fever pitch, and there was a period of about three to six months where, outside of school, I would not leave the safety of my home, for there was nothing out there in town and the surrounding area for me to do, not if it meant running into the wrong people or being alone in my activities. My parents did their best to try to help me, but my continued denial of autism, the need to put the blame on others, and the belief that my parents could not possibly understand what I was going through prevented any kind of assistance or breakthroughs from taking place. This often led to many arguments and confrontations, with my mother trying to use tough love and to show me the need to face the reality of my condition. Instead of toughening my skin, it only made me retreat further into myself and become my insecurities, as I felt that her confrontational approach was little more than beating me into submission. As for my father, while he took a far more sensitive and delicate approach, he put his faith in autism experts and other professionals instead of his own ability to bond with me and attempt to understand my confused and vulnerable psyche; my denials and belief that he knew nothing of my struggle did not help either. My brother Nick initially knew nothing about my condition. which I had intended from the day I was diagnosed, but when the truth eventually came out he tended to stay out of these fights, partially because I wanted him too but also because he felt it was easier to focus on his own life. As much as I wish he could have been there for me the way I tried to be for him as his big brother, deep down I knew it was better that he remained disconnected from my struggles and denials about my condition, especially when he said he did not want to understand it or have anything to do with it.

So, I threw myself into my schoolwork and my work at the theater, the intensity of which aggravated my already despairing state and began developing into a cocktail of high stress, anxiety, and depression. I had isolated myself, creating a series of islands to shelter from the storms and cyclones that were wreaking havoc on my entire life, rowing between them through the storms and getting done what needed to be done before moving on. Sometimes these islands would be television and video games where often, in my lowest moments, the pixelated characters on the screens served as the only real friends I had. Two other occasions further justified my situation, with the latter convincing me to fight back against the reign of terror I faced. The friend I still had, M. A., a tall, athletic girl I had known since middle school who went to another school where she was a basketball champion, had been a faithful friend and confidante for years. All of a sudden she disappeared from my life, refusing to answer my calls, and her friends shunned me when I asked what was going on. This genuine confusion and cluelessness would last for a long time until I finally realized it was because my stress and anxiety fueled a lack of self-awareness in her life, and those feelings proved too much for her to cope with.

The second occasion put my life in danger. At seventeen, having built up so much anxiety and stress that I was terrified at the thought of securing my driver's license, I was riding my bike the five-mile distance between work and home. The hardest part was pushing myself to pedal up the last half mile of hillside that separated me from my house. I was halfway up when I heard the sound of a car engine heading downhill toward me. As always, I moved to the side of the road while continuing to pedal upward, confident that I would have enough room to continue forward like I had many times before. The car was hard to miss: a large white Chevrolet Suburban SUV with a gleaming silver grille fixed over the engine right above the front bumper. From the front it seemed to fill a significant portion of the street as it rounded a corner about a hundred yards ahead of me. However, it was not the car I focused on the most; it was the driver and the passengers who sat beside him. At that moment, I was in big trouble.

The boy driving it was not just any boy; M.S. was one of the most popular kids in school, coming from a multimillionaire family with a history of being the best in local sports. To me, however, he was huge, threatening, and thuggish. If there was anyone who was presiding over the ruling elite of my high school, pulling the strings and waving his wallet around, it was him. A year before, I was riding the same bike to work from school and as I passed by him on the sidewalk, he laughed at my bike, shook his car keys at me, and gloatingly shouted that he was about to climb into his new car. Now, that car was barreling down the narrow, winding road, and he had just spotted me coming toward them. The moment felt almost suspended in time; it was as if I could read his thoughts, see the gears working in his mind, and watch the reaction on his heavy face, in his bulging green eyes. His reaction was one of pure, gleeful dominance—and one of instilling terror. The screech of rubber on pavement pierced the quiet neighborhood as the SUV's tires were turned to my right and the car itself turned left to the edge of the road, almost running through the gutter that made up the shoulder, blocking the entire stretch of pavement, and filling my vision with the sight of steel and glass that most likely weighed about three tons and was moving at around thirty miles an hour. A loud and explicit swear word rushed past my lips as I realized I had nowhere to run and nowhere near enough time to get out of the way of the hulking metallic entity that I believed was about to run me over. Another screech once again filled the air, and the SUV turned back onto the road, missing me and my bike, although the side mirror almost grazed my head and the force of the wind that the car carried nearly knocked me to the ground. I swore I heard a shout of derisive laughter from inside the car before it disappeared around the corner and out of sight.

With extreme difficulty, I was able to haul my numb body the last three hundred yards to the driveway and up the thirty steps to the front door of my house, at which point I called my father and told him what had happened. Agreeing that this had finally gone too far, he promptly called the boy's father, told them what had happened, and threatened police action if they did not ensure that they put him in his place. While initially defensive of his son and offhandedly citing his athletic ability, he eventually agreed to tell M.S. to never pull a dangerous stunt like that again and to stay away from me.

That event was the peak moment in the long line of systemic social abuse, neglect, and betrayal I had received at the hands of my peers over the years, and I could not allow it to continue. I decided that something had to change. I already had a strong work ethic, had found other interests to pursue, and had a potential for seeking an untapped market of opportunities. I was not going to allow a small town of shallow, corrupt, and self-possessed people to drag me down any further, nor would I allow my rage and defensive nature to sink my worth down to their level. I promised myself that I would be better, braver, and more ready to take on whatever came next, and soon, I would rise above all of the despair and dysfunction that had held me back for so long. While my social life and existence within the community had been taken away from me by their heinous actions, they would not take away the rest of my life.

INTERLUDE
REFLECTION AND SELF-INTROSPECTION

"Don't forget that I cannot see myself, that my role is limited to being the one who looks in the mirror."
— Jacques Rigaut

A monologue of one's life can either draw in a crowd or bore them to tears. The story needs to have substance and a means to hook the attention of the masses and a central character that readers feel for and want to rally around. Readers need to feel the experiences as that person did, to know what it was like, and, of course, to know how to avoid experiencing unpleasant issues in their lives and prepare for the inevitable. For many people who have lived extraordinary lives, who either created an original idea that positively affected many or who managed to overcome unthinkable adversity, those are the individuals that people hold onto. I am not one of those people.

I have never considered myself to be extraordinary, nor have I come up with truly original ideas to better humanity. I am someone who considered myself to be normal but was treated as anything but normal. I am someone who wanted to make a positive difference, original or otherwise, in whatever way I could, and who had the willpower and determination to do it, but faced a more determined opposition intent on derailing me at any cost. Furthermore, I was someone who was convinced for a long time that I understood and could be like all the other people I grew up with, without sacrificing who I was as an individual. I was oblivious to the fact that they never saw me as one of them and what they did not understand resulted in acts of fear and cruelty toward me. It took me years to understand all of this, long after the facts of my early life had been established.

The reasons, in reality, were quite simple: my wall of denial and my being unaware that I genuinely lacked understanding of social situations. Essentially, I believed I had a stronger moral compass, more maturity, a better distinction between right and wrong, more passion in my interests and a stronger work ethic than most people I knew at my age, but my overall social development was off and grew at a slower pace than others I interacted with.

In addition to slowed social growth, there were also parts of normal social development that I either did not possess or had not been able to learn yet because of my inability to process social events normally. A key example is how easy it was for me to constantly forget to check, much less be aware of, the nonverbal cues and facial expressions people showed when I was talking to them. In hindsight, that would most likely have been a factor into why some people, such as my erstwhile best friend or any of the girls I wanted to be romantically involved with, felt uncomfortable around me and sometimes reacted badly.

It was, and still is, difficult for me to inject myself into a conversation I was either a small part of or not part of at all; in addition, I have felt compelled to finish my position in a conversation, oblivious to the change and flow within it, feeling a compulsive need to complete my thought. In that scenario, often in school and free time, I could have appeared as socially awkward and withdrawn, as well as controlling, due to my need to finish and/or defend my positions. Impulse control was then, and sometimes still is, an issue that makes me think that while I was growing up, I did things that felt right and completely normal but, from the reactions of others, turned out not to be (*how I talked, the tone of my voice, how I approached others, etc.*), hence furthering an image of a weird and potentially disturbing individual. While it is possible that my autism came with an acute reaction to stress, anxiety, and depression, I stand by my assertion that my experiences in the years following my diagnosis served only to heighten my emotional responses and ingrain them into my psyche, shaping them into a force powerful enough to give the impression that they had a mind of their own and could occur at any time in any place, with me being powerless to stop it.

Sure enough, whenever there was a subject I did not understand or when I was forced to do new things and prepare to be a busy and responsible adult, these emotions were quick to take over and cloud my judgment often to the point of inaction. For example, this explains why it took so long for me to obtain a driver's license and why I would often have knee-jerk reactions to sudden changes in my work environment if routines were broken or new, unfamiliar responsibilities were given. The effect of these changes, coupled with my social/academic issues and pressures, affected my depression. There were a great many reasons for my situational depression, and as the episodes became more numerous and intense, they had an effect similar to seizures: once they started, there was absolutely no stopping them, and the only thing that could be done was to ride them out until they dissipated.

Despite these extraordinarily common and intense emotional episodes, and the feeling that there was no way out of my circumstances, I never truly got to the point where, like so many unfortunate teenagers, I seriously considered suicide. While I will admit that there was a brief moment where I pondered whether the world would be better off without me, in the end I realized that I was far more afraid of death than the possibility of living and feeling like I had a life worse than death. There was also the fact that in addition to valuing my life, my family, coworkers, and mentors throughout my childhood and adolescence valued it even more because they saw someone worthy of love, attention and compassion. When the day came that I decided to take back control of my life, I would finally be able to see a way forward and, soon enough, the light waiting for me at the end of the long tunnel I had wandered through for so long.

CHAPTER 9
SALVATION LIES WITHIN

The choice was made, but the seed had already been planted years before. Parallel to all of the disparity and difficult situations I had ever faced, there was another path being created that would not only assist in my maturity into adulthood but give me hope that there was a good future for me at the end of it. Like the trials and tribulations I was facing, this path was built by the same accumulation of experiences, but it resided strictly within the realm of positivity. While I had the support and understanding of the upperclassmen at school, as well as the support system of my family and some teachers, it was not enough, and that motivated me to further branch out and build a bigger community for myself, which in turn led me to seek interests outside of the town that had held me back for so long.

My original desire to make money through recycling had already transformed into a full-fledged interest in environmental work, which led me to pursue employment in that field. As a result, with the support and guidance of my parents, I found and was accepted into an internship at the University of California, Berkeley, at the age of fifteen. This internship, the TEAMS (*Teens Exploring and Achieving in Math and Science*) program, introduced me to more advanced methods of learning, thinking, and teaching in the realm of environmental work, as well as opening a gate to the rest of the San Francisco Bay area. Through this program I made friends from all corners of the Bay, and they were a diverse group compared with the mostly Caucasian community I had come from. Every one of them had a fascinating background in terms of experience, culture, and racial makeup, which led to my interest in understanding people from those backgrounds. This, in turn, taught me two things: they were not only different in their experiences and cultures, but they were the same as me, in the sense that we all wanted both a professional experience in this internship and the opportunity to expand our thinking and understanding of each other, thereby creating a community and many new friends in the process.

In the three years that I had this internship, my interest in environmentalism and my desire to have a broader group of friends continued to grow. I learned many professional skills in the various tasks I was given, the most prominent being the work I did in the biology education lab, which educated children about various animal species and their importance to the natural world. As someone who was obsessed with animals when I was their age, it was a good way for me to give back to the community and assist in their education. I also learned how to balance the act of bonding with the children while keeping up professional appearances in how I handled myself with the animals and my interactions with the students and their parents. In addition to my work in the lab, I participated in various community projects, one of which saw me and my fellow interns restoring a major creek bed that ran through various East Bay Area communities that had been affected by both soil erosion and damage from societal activities (*trash, vandalism, industrial pollution, etc.*). One of my internship favorites occurred every summer, when I volunteered to join a coastal ecology camp in the Santa Cruz mountains as a counselor for kids aged eight to twelve. During the three summers that I volunteered there, I learned the value of teaching in an environment far removed from my comfort zone, as well as responsibility for the kids I was put in charge of. This transformative experience came from the realization that I could be both a mentor to them and a superior that kept them in line and on their best behavior. These kids needed someone to look up to and guide them, and because of that, I saw this as an opportunity to be the kind of supporting figure that was there for them the way that so many back home were not there for me.

My personal growth also came from the interactions with my colleagues, who knew what it was like to come from different backgrounds and be treated differently and, as a result, we leaned on each other for support. Through this solidarity, we were able to do and accomplish many things together, for example, putting on a campfire skit for the kids and joining my father on his sailboat in the San Francisco Bay to celebrate my birthday, thereby breaking a personal cycle where my birthday was, for a number of years, just a quiet family affair with no one else home to celebrate with. The best part about this was the fact that they neither noticed nor cared that I was not as socially adept as they were, for their inclusive nature and their tendency to come up with various humorous antics to generate a fun and light-hearted atmosphere gave me such a feeling of ease that I almost never had to worry about how I acted around them, nor did I have to think too much about what they thought of me. The many professional and personal accomplishments I made contributed to my overall confidence and the belief that there was more opportunity out there for me. All I had to do was go out there and seize it.

Opportunities came in ways that I least expected. Shortly after starting my internship, and not long after my sixteenth birthday, I got my first real job (*because of my former friend Z.M.*) at the movie theater, where I was able to further solidify the strong work ethic I had already been developing at my internship. The managerial staff, while corporate-minded and mostly caring about the bottom line, nonetheless saw my commitment and willingness to do what needed to be done, and as such, always had plenty of work for me to do and allowed me to get as much experience as allowed for a minor like me. In addition, I also had certain privileges like seeing movies for free. During one of my shifts I became captivated by a movie involving urban street dance, more commonly known as "hip-hop." After I used my privileges to see the movie in its entirety, it was as if something turned on a light inside me I did not even know I had. I did not know it then, but my entire perspective in life changed after seeing that film. What I saw was not just a series of choreographed routines, but a story of people who had gone through tough times of varying degrees, yet were able to come together and create something special with nothing but their wits, bodies, and collective will to make it happen. Those themes, including the diversity and the real-life connotations to the dance community at large, encouraged me to seek out further opportunities than what I had already found.

Through viewing reality competitions of hip-hop dance and seeking out dance workshops to learn the various dance styles that were offered, I not only became a proficient recreational dancer, but I also discovered another, very inclusive, community of people who accepted me as I was and allowed for me to grow as an individual alongside them. In addition, I discovered my passion for altruistic work involving the mentoring of young, underprivileged children and helping to feed the impoverished residents of towns and municipalities in the Southern Bay Area. I often worked alongside my fellow dancers whom, while holding a high status in those communities because of their work, nonetheless never forgot their humble beginnings and roots in those places and made it their mission to give back however they could.

The third and biggest surprise for me was taking on a passion passed down by my parents. Through my connections to various environmental groups, I discovered an organization known as the Green Screen, a group of teenagers like myself who ran an independently operated television program broadcast throughout the Bay Area. Having already proved myself as a proficient writer in school, and curious to see what the media industry had been like for my parents, I reached out to the director of Green Screen. My "interview" consisted of my doing a field report at a party ahead of an awards ceremony for high school–aged individuals who were chosen for environmental projects they created that had national and international effects and exposure. In my interviews, I not only met many inspirational people, but I also discovered I was just as good at engaging in professional conversation as I was at writing about events and people. With the success of my coverage of that event, I was promptly hired and was brought into a team consisting of about fifteen people of various technical and reporting skills. Most of the team came from the northern Bay Area town of Richmond, which was (*and still is*) a town situated next to a major oil refinery and is home to a number of poor, mostly minority residents. Through my work with the Green Screen, I not only saw my face on many of the local networks, but in addition to the stories I told for hundreds of thousands across the region, I also got involved with many of the local residents and their environmental projects. These exposures through my job further cemented my belief that I was doing worthwhile work, and they broadened my horizons and perspective on just how multifaceted the world of environmentalism was, including the correlation between preserving natural habitats and the effect pollution and lack of resources had on poor communities.

By the time I had reached my senior year in high school, I was working three jobs. Every one of them was a paying job, but each a different caliber: my work at the cinema was a typical hourly wage job akin to many private sector entry-level jobs, my internship was a paid one based on a fixed amount for every weekend I worked, and my job as an environmental news reporter was a fixed monthly stipend. While they did not amount to a lot of money individually, together they helped me build a small fortune, at least in the eyes of someone who was about to cross the threshold into college. They also made me feel good about myself compared with many of my trust fund classmates who eventually had to find summer jobs before college as their way of learning responsibility. Altogether, these jobs and the communities I became a part of in the process elevated me above the daily issues, insults, and difficult situations I constantly found myself in at school and in the suburban bubble that was the town of Lafayette.

One final encounter helped me reclaim much of my glass-completely-full attitude. While at a dance workshop in the southern Bay Area town of Hayward, I discovered that one of the guest teachers was a prominent Hollywood dancer named Taeko McCarroll. For me, this was one of the first instances where I experienced a Forrest Gump–like encounter the way my parents did in their journalism professions decades ago: Taeko was a true hip-hop dancer, with a tough-as-nails attitude when it came to making it in the Hollywood entertainment industry and passing on her knowledge and skills to others. She also happened to be of Japanese descent, which I took advantage of by greeting her in Japanese and briefly letting her know of my birth in Japan and the influence of Japanese culture (*food, pop culture, artifacts in my home*) in my life. While our connection did not officially start with that encounter and taking her workshop, we stayed in touch over a number of months until I convinced her of my journalist skills and background and offered to assist her in a dance culture news blog affectionately named Koifysh.com that she made to shine a light on the events and effects of the broader dance community.

For years after that, I would tell my family and friends, old and new, that she was one of the few people who gave me a chance when almost no one else would. I started out as a media researcher, finding stories and making connections and deals with other dancers to send me stories of their own exploits. Within only a few months, I went from local dance stories to a nationwide web of various people, dance crews, companies, studios, and events, even going as far as posting a story about a group of Canadian dancers who put on a show for the Queen of England. Impressed with my initiative and demonstrated ability to greatly expand her blog, Taeko promoted me to co-manage the blog with her, which involved me providing direct oversight of all information on it, especially when she was preoccupied with other matters in the dance industry. For me, this promotion was not only one of the highlights of my young life, but also the final piece of the puzzle that comprised the connections, jobs, friends, and community I had managed to single-handedly build up for myself.

Through it all, however, I continued to deny my autism and kept the taboo in place, and every time my parents attempted to bring it up in discussions about my troubles at school, I would promptly shut them down and continue to blame others for the suffering I was still enduring. Perhaps it was due to the success of my work and my personal and professional relationships that I continued to persuade myself that I was a normal person after all. In one of my more vulnerable periods, I had learned that those not affected by autism were known as neurotypical, or "normal-brained," people with no issues in socializing whatsoever. In addition, certain people in my life who knew or figured out what my disorder was tried to assure me that everyone has problems with socializing and understanding people. In hindsight, I realize that they were trying to make me feel better and less self-conscious of myself, but at the time it only served to confuse me more. For if everyone had that issue, why was I always standing out, and if they, for the most part, were having an easier time establishing relationships with others and socializing at consistent rates, why was I still relegated to just my work and the infrequent social encounters I had with my friends around the Bay Area?

Despite these questions, I turned my focus to preparing for my first year at San Francisco State University. With the success of my jobs and volunteer work, and my adolescent woes seemingly in my rearview mirror, I crossed the Bay Bridge onto a new adventure, hopeful and determined to become a better, more mature person and begin to cement a functioning, independent life on a journey toward full, realized adulthood. A fresh start was on the horizon, and it would turn autism and everything associated with it into a distant memory, or so I wanted to believe.

STAGE TWO

YOUNG ADULTHOOD

"What lies behind us and what lies before us are tiny matters compared to what lies within us."

— Ralph Waldo Emerson

CHAPTER 10
IT FOLLOWS

There are more than seven wonders of the world, more wonders than I believe anyone can truly comprehend. For me, the wonders are things that astound you when you least expect it, sometimes involving things that you have already seen but have not truly appreciated until a certain point. I had always been aware of and had experienced San Francisco, but for the first time in my life, I was actually going to live there on my own. Crossing that bridge, seeing the skyline of downtown, the red and white of the distant Sutro Tower, and the picturesque bay that contained Alcatraz and Angel Island, the Golden Gate Bridge, and the distant Marin Headlands, I relaxed for the first time in years and quickly convinced myself that this new chapter of my life would usher in a new era of improvement and stability for me, the chance to start over again.

Before I left for college, I promised myself to purge as much of my existence in Lafayette as possible, starting with cleansing myself of my horrific experiences and most of the people I knew there. I put yearbooks into storage, wiped my social media clean of my time there, and cut ties with everyone whom I believed did not deserve a place in my future (*mostly my tormentors and their friends*), all the while packing most of my possessions to move into my new dormitory. There was, of course, no ridding myself of the memories of what I had faced, but with renewed optimism and a new life ahead of me, it was enough for me to push all that into a small corner of my mind. I looked forward to the creation of new memories and experiences, and hopefully I could create a safe haven of sorts so I would not feel as if anything had followed me there.

Familiar things can sneak up on you. At first, the feeling of starting over and being a new person can be all-consuming. I quickly made new friends, including a boy named A.K., a short, robust Filipino with a long and messy mop of black hair whom I met at orientation and who hailed from the northern California town of Chico. He quickly became a close friend, even while in a different dormitory on the other side of campus. With the start of the first week of college, it was all about becoming familiar with the new college scene. People from all walks of life joined our group, from my three roommates to the many other people who frequented my on-campus apartment for social gatherings and illegal drinks. Some hailed from the other end of the state, others were from immigrant families, and still more were of different political opinions (*socialist to conservative*) and sexual orientations (*homosexual to nonbinary*). I met a girl named K.D., who at first glance was an attractive young Korean-American woman with whom I got along very well. As I quickly discovered, however, attractive young women were exactly the kind of people she liked and wanted to date. That experience taught me two things: I should not assume anything about a person and their interests, and despite my initial feelings for her, I was able to transform them into a strong bond of friendship over the course of that year, as she proved herself to be a nice, trusting, and dependable friend.

While these improvements were being made, however, familiar feelings also began creeping back into my life: stress, anxiety, and depression. The first two reappeared as I was learning two important things about college life: I must do better in academics than I ever did in high school (*which, at barely a 3.1 GPA, was not very good for an honors-oriented school and having a less-than-helpful teaching staff, most of whom had written me off an average student*), and I had to find a balance between my blossoming social life and studies. The first year of college was not a success story in that regard. Furthermore, my maternal grandfather passed away shortly after the school year began, which brought about an extended period of depression, though in this case, I had support from A.K. and the new friends we had made together. Despite this, unconsciously, I regressed into the kind of person who prioritized his academics above everything else. I needed a space where I felt comfortable enough to do my work and feel less pressure and distraction, and so this resulted in my riding the train thirty miles back home nearly every weekend to my family and to my comfort zone. While it did lead to a surge in my grade point average like I had never known before, it also carried the price of keeping me away from many of the friends I had made. It further built the image of a young man who was only viewing himself as a student, nothing more.

Recognizing and accepting the problem did not make it go away so easily. I still wanted to have the kind of social life that had eluded me for so long, and I attempted to make an effort to achieve that end. I joined hip-hop dance classes with A.K., underwent fitness training at the campus gym, and continued to familiarize myself with the broader community, on and off campus. As I did so, however, I began to find myself in newer, but no less difficult, social situations. A prominent example was when I was getting to know A.K. and his girlfriend, D.D., a high school student he had left in Chico. During the first semester of college, two things happened simultaneously: A.K. began to show impatience with me as well as criticism of my flaws, and D.D. began to withdraw from him when he showed the same kind of emotional abuse to her. As a result, she turned to me for comfort. Tolerant and caring soul that I was and trusting her for having been there for me when my grandfather passed, we leaned on each other for emotional support, until the day D.D. told me she had a major crush on me. It was as if my mind had split in two; one side was saying that I should take advantage of the fact that for the first time a girl with long dirty-blonde hair and the face and body of a Victoria's Secret model outwardly admitted feelings for me, while the other side told me it was the worst thing to consider, for I should not return the feeling as long as she was with someone else. I decided on a compromise: I told her I felt the same way, but made it clear that it could never happen as long as she was with A.K., but that I would not let her continue to be abused and not have someone to talk to.

For a time, it seemed to work. We talked whenever we felt sad and needed someone to cheer us up, and it turned out we also shared an interest in dance. I was always careful never to cross the line and act on those feelings that would break every rule and boundary regarding established relationships. In addition, I wanted to repair my friendship with A.K., but it soon became apparent that he was descending into a dark place on his own as he escalated his behavior toward me. The biggest escalation was when I was walking to class and received a message from him. We had a minor fight the night before, in which he nonspecifically stated that he was not sure if we were healthy for each other as friends and that it probably would not work out. I thought I had succeeded in convincing him that he was acting impulsively, that we were only through our first semester, and we just needed to be there for each other no matter the struggles in order for our friendship to succeed.

The message he sent the next day derailed all hopes of that happening. In the first of what turned into a fiery stream of messages, he called me out as an incompetent, annoying, and, above all, creeper of a human being who was all around "deaf and blind," didn't know how to bond with others, and whose attitude and actions chased everyone away. He finished by saying that I deserved to be alone and that the people we met together, who I called my friends, were secretly weirded out and afraid of me because of my personality and strange habits. I responded by warning him not to say anything more unless he wanted me to turn these messages over to the campus police department. The response worked, and he desisted from all further communication. In addition, I was further dismayed when, despite not defending his behavior, D.D. chose to stay with him. She decided it was only going to hurt me to stay in touch with her, which resulted in my breaking off our connection as well. I would find out the next year that A.K. had dropped out of college and went home, where he attempted to reconcile with her, only for that to fail and for him to end up joining the military. Subsequently, I reconnected with her twice more over the years, only to discover that she could not grow out of her immature, small-town attitude and her lack of commitment to us when we had the chance forced me to permanently cut ties with her.

Dismayed as I was with them and the hurtful rhetoric A.K. had used, I took comfort in realizing that none of what he said was true. When I approached the other friends I had made when A.K. and I were still on good terms, they affirmed that they liked me very much, with one of them relating to me on how she used to be "walked all over," socially speaking, by others at her former high school. While I did not end up being as close to them as I wanted to over the course of my schooling, with a few of them leaving and/or transferring to other schools over time, I considered this to be a victory, knowing that this was only an isolated incident of animosity toward me and I had actually been able to read the others by their actions and rhetoric to know that they thought well of me and my character. There were too few people in high school who had seen me this way and many more who had treated me with similar animosity, reinforcing my belief in an improvement by comparison.

Even so, as I continued to advance in both academics and relationships with my classmates and other students, I still felt out of place. Part of that feeling came from how my anxiety, in addition to the pressures of academia, also affected my anticipation of social interactions, which led to extreme self-consciousness and a constant stream of second-guessing if I was doing things right. From my perspective, it appeared that whether it was making a friend, finding a love interest, getting an invite to a party, or just attempting to make friendly conversation, there was an X factor that everyone else had, men and women alike, that I did not, and I could never figure out what that winning formula was. As this continued on throughout my first year, I finally decided I needed answers, some way to figure out how to chart a course through this quagmire of shifting social cues and atmosphere. With that decision, a small crack appeared in the wall, and small pieces began falling away as it slowly started to crumble.

CHAPTER 11
THE FIRST STEP

In my experience, there is hardly ever one moment in time, a sudden spark of realization, or an epiphany out of the blue, that propels you to do something you never considered doing in the first place. A series of factors led to me finally seeking help for my condition, the first being a presentation I gave in my communications class during my freshman year. We were to give individual informative presentations on something that either interested us or meant the most to us and express it to our classmates. One of the students gave a presentation in which he made a very personal admission to the entire class: he was a high-functioning autistic individual. He described what made him different from the rest of us and why he was still proud to think of himself as someone who could still live his life and accept his various behavioral differences as normal without public perception interfering. To help us understand, he passed out a slip of paper that broke down the distinct differences between individuals afflicted with autism and individuals with neurotypical brains. I read through them, taking note that more than half of the symptoms did not apply to me, which included the need for strict routines, having narrow interests, and not showing emotions at the appropriate times. I did, however, correspond to increased sensitivity to loud noise, difficulty with accepting change, and having acute stressors compared with the average neurotypical.

Having it all laid out in front of me forced me to face the fact that while I was not severely autistic, I was nonetheless on the spectrum, if only slightly. Perhaps it was watching a person my age openly admitting and embracing his autism, or seeing the facts before me instead of dictated to by a psychiatrist, that began to soften the way I saw myself and how I had initially looked at my diagnosis. After class, my classmate, Eli Agustin, and I were walking around campus together talking about the emotional weight of the presentations, including the one on autism, and I decided to be brave and tell her that it affected me because I am also on the spectrum. She looked at me with such a kind face slightly curtained by her long brown hair, and instead of my seeing a look of distaste, embarrassment, or discomfort, her soft brown eyes shone with wonder, surprise, and realization. She told me that she really appreciated honesty and that even her "normal" friends were often incapable of being as open with her as I was. She further stated that she was glad it was in my nature to be such a kind, considerate, and open individual. With her words and the feeling like a great weight had been lifted off my shoulders, I decided that if I truly wanted to feel more accepting of myself, I needed to at least consider the need for professional help so I could better understand myself and how I could bond with others more effectively.

I began seeing a therapist who, after hearing me describe myself and the affliction I dealt with on a regular basis, directed me to group therapy where I could hear others describe their struggles at being accepted in society and accepting themselves in the process. To me, some of them were a bit unremarkable, such as the one who was being judged for having a tough, mean-looking persona and was reinforcing the stereotype by lashing out in frustration. But one person, H.X., described the inner turmoil she felt when it came to viewing herself and how she must look in the eyes of so many others. In addition she felt depressed, anxious, and alone, sometimes for no reason. As she spoke, the emotion in her face was so genuine that I began to feel all of her feelings. Not wanting her to continue being in pain and seeing her eyes welling with so many tears, I gave her a reassuring hug while promising her she was not alone and I would be right by her side. When the session was over, H.X. approached me and told me that while she normally did not like to be touched by a person she just met, she nonetheless felt safe and reassured by my act of selflessness and understanding. We became friends shortly after, and while I stopped going to the session several months later, feeling they were not addressing me as an autistic individual, we remained in touch and spent more time together. She eventually departed for school in Santa Barbara, but not before reminding me that I was more than the sum of my insecurities and could be a stronger and better person if I believed that. I want to say that her advice worked, but the sum of my insecurities was much more than even she could comprehend and would continue to be a challenge going forward.

In the latter half of my freshman year I joined a class that was considered unique to the entire American university system: A Hip-Hop Workshop. This workshop was dedicated to the entire counterculture that hip-hop is, with everything from the inner workings of the rap music industry to how the various hip-hop forms (rapping, graffiti, dancing, etc.) were being used to make statements for social change. It was one of the most fascinating classes I had ever taken and would ever take in college, and was made even more enjoyable when we were told that our final had to be a group presentation on persuading the professors, the class, and a group of hip-hop auditors from out of state to see hip-hop as an integral part of certain societal systems. My group was chosen to explain how hip-hop and education are of equal importance and therefore should be taught together. When the day arrived, my group put together a presentation where we would each describe a different slide, ending with me highlighting the importance of hip-hop and education being considered one and the same. When it came time for me to speak, I was nervous, especially since I was in front of well over 150 people, but in that moment, I decided to let the nerves mix with my confidence and just let the energy flow. What followed was a high-powered presentation where I articulated how certain education programs like the arts were being slashed from school budgets and put aside much the way hip-hop was also being disregarded by those in upper mainstream society, and how we have a responsibility to our communities and our children to give them these opportunities to learn the "street smarts and the book smarts" so that they will aspire to be good citizens and human beings.

All at once, like a giant wave about to break and crash on the shore, the entire audience got up and gave an enormous round of applause, with plenty of cheering and whistling in between all of the clapping. I had not heard a sound nor seen a spectacle like that since my disastrous run for student body vice president in high school, only this time I could tell that the applause and cheering was genuine. When it finally died down and our professors began giving their judgments, one of them looked at me and asked if I was planning to run for governor. He said it sounded as if I was trying to get everyone to vote for me so I could be the one to make this proposal a reality, which went to show how passionate I was and what this subject meant to me. The only thing better than subsequently getting a perfect score on my final was the gratitude I felt for everyone who believed I had done an incredible job and the realization that I had a talent for public speaking. From that point on, whenever it came to classes and events that involved speaking in front of everyone and where the subject matter was important to me, I flourished in that environment, and for the most part, my social ineptitudes never caused any problems for me when I was speaking in a public setting as opposed to a few people in a private one. As freshman year came to an end, and I had to pack up and move back home for the summer, for the first time in a long time I looked forward to whatever came next, even more so than I had dared hoped when the year had first begun. My figurative glass was starting to become full again, alongside the cracked foundations in the wall of denial that once held so strong.

CHAPTER 12
PHOENIX RISING

The islands of my life had begun to rise out of the stormy seas, transforming into land masses that were holding steady amid the beatings the water still gave it on a constant basis. The rest of my time in college had slowly begun to shape into the kind of life I had always wanted for myself, though with a constant reminder that I had to be wary of how it could change at any time, giving me more of a reason to maintain a balance in both my social and academic life. Even with the continued presence of stress and anxiety, the constant amount of schoolwork, and the need to be aware and alert for the unexpected (*a serious example being when I missed the deadline for a semester's worth of classes because the reminder for fees ended up in my junk email and took weeks of bureaucracy to get the classes back*), I still found ways to thoroughly enjoy my time on and off campus. My circle of friends had grown as I moved to new apartments every year with new roommates and new avenues in the social realm. I continued attending hip-hop dance classes, taking part in campus activities like Occupy Wall Street protests fighting for economic equality and an end to crushing student debt, and maintaining focus in most of my classes. One of my crowning achievements in academia was how I ended up on the dean's list for seven of my eight semesters of college, as this honor was given to few students and filled me with pride and happiness knowing that I was not the average student that many of my high school teachers and counselors had written me off to be.

I was beginning to prepare myself for professional work after graduation, while also finding opportunities that resulted in life-changing experiences, shaping my perspective in such a way that I knew what I stood for and wanted to do for the rest of my life. The summer after my freshman year, I was given what I believed to be two golden opportunities: a reporting assignment for Taeko McCarroll's dance blog in Hollywood for the show America's Best Dance Crew, followed by an internship at the office of the district attorney for the East Bay county of Contra Costa. Flying into Los Angeles felt like a dream, for while I had family and friends in the city and had visited many times before, this was the first time I was going there to work a real assignment for a Hollywood dancer on a show that I had been a fan of for years that was filmed at Warner Bros. Studios.

The surreal experience continued as I went through the motions of warming up for interviews; got an official press pass to enter the studio; saw the intricate arrangements of the central stage, the surrounding stands, and the press lounge; and of course, saw the dancers and Hollywood moguls that made this show a reality. Meeting Randy Jackson of American Idol fame was quite an experience. Despite being my father's age, he acted a lot more like my nineteen-year-old self, which only made him that much more fun and interesting as an individual. While I did not get a lot of time with him, I got to know his partner in the show's creation a lot more. Howard Schwartz was an upstanding middle-aged gentleman who believed in the innovation of reality television, as well as allowing dancers, particularly hip-hop dancers, to have more of the spotlight that is usually reserved for singers and actors. After interviewing him, I told him of how this show inspired me to want to both dance and to support the dance community however I could, having already done so much for the Bay Area dance community and wanting to take it to the next level. In turn, he asked me to attend Hip Hop International, a competition he created eight years before, so I could get to know the international community and see what they do for dance and each other. When it came to interviewing the dancers who hailed from all corners of the United States, I felt immediate kinship with them, which forced me to make a bit of an effort to maintain objectivity as a reporter. The two weeks I spent in Los Angeles ended up as a success in two ways, as I successfully filmed interviews with many prominent dancers and entertainment officials and I got to know the community more intimately than I ever could have imagined.

Shortly after my time in Hollywood, I arrived home to start my internship working for the district attorney. My job consisted of working alongside other interns, precisely filing various cases that ranged from drunk driving to domestic abuse, while occasionally sitting in on county court trials to observe the proceedings. I was partially inspired to undertake this internship because my mother was a lawyer and had recently started working in the field of elder law, in addition to always having a curiosity for how the American legal system worked and having a friend whose father was a county judge. In my time there I made friends among the interns I worked with and also made an impression on various lawyers and prosecutors, including the deputy district attorney (DDA). One impression in particular occurred when we were witnessing a trial where the DDA herself was the prosecutor and was bringing forward a case against a soldier who allegedly resisted arrest and committed battery against a police officer while he and his girlfriend were being questioned in a suspicious driving incident. The trial lasted several days, during which I followed and documented as much of the process as possible. Before the jury reached a verdict, my fellow interns and I were individually interviewed by the DDA and asked what our observations of the proceedings were.

In great detail, I described to her how I believed the defendant was quietly furious at the proceedings, fully believing himself to be innocent of all charges. When character witnesses were called and described him in an unsavory way, he interrupted the proceedings in an aggressive manner that caused the judge to send the jury out of the room and to reprimand him for his behavior. Furthermore, I stated that with such an aggressive demeanor and the fact that he dishonored the court by wearing his army uniform for a civilian court proceeding (*the military expects uniforms to be worn for military court martials only*) I believed him to be guilty of one, possibly both charges. It was the best guess I could give her because that was the only conclusion I could come up with from what I saw in that courtroom. After a few seconds of silence, she humorously asked me if I was considering a career in sports commentating, highlighting how articulate I was in describing the proceedings and that I had a real talent for observing everything said and done around me. This was the second time I had heard someone in a position of power be so impressed with me that they could see me going on to do great things. Even more surprising to me was her comment on my observational skills, seeing as social cues and reading behavior was not my strong suit as an autistic person. From then on I continued to do well in my summer internship, though the difference now was that I felt even more empowered and confident professionally and socially.

My social life began to take on a new tone. Having made many friends in the local dance community and learning about and from people who lived a life very different than mine, I began to bond with them to the point that, in one prominent instance, I brought one friend from my old life in Lafayette into the life I now had that crisscrossed the greater Bay Area. S.S., one of my two best friends from middle school and onward, was the only friend left from my youth now that Z.M. was officially out of the picture. He had been attending school in Southern California for the past two years but had recently come back to reconsider his options. During that time I invited him to a party in Castro Valley, located in the southern Bay Area. Many of my friends from the dance community lived there, and one of them was throwing the party, which happened to be a birthday party for him and two of his friends who shared the same day.

We drove down together, I introduced him to everyone, and for what can only be described as five hours of absolute fun and excitement, S.S. and I thoroughly enjoyed our time getting to know people who lived different lives from us and who possessed different attitudes involving open arms, an appreciation of different people, and all-around acceptance—in addition to great music, dance, and drinks. As we drove away from Castro Valley, S.S. told me that the party was the best one he had ever been to, describing how the parties he had been to back in Lafayette and down in Southern California involved a lot of "fake" people who didn't care much about others and more about themselves, their image, and whatever kind of hedonistic benefits they could get out of it. His admission made me feel that not only had I made the right friends, but that I had opened him up to a better world beyond the bubble that was Lafayette and the surrounding communities that looked inward instead of outward at the diversity and acceptance of the San Francisco Bay Area.

CHAPTER 13
PEAK SENSATION

Hollywood had all of the glitz, glamor, and opportunities, and the district attorney's office had its share of interesting cases and strivers I worked alongside, but to think that this would be as good as it got for me could not be further from the truth. Beginning in my sophomore year of college, I became a more serious activist involved in many different social justice causes, the most prominent being a rapidly expanding campaign by the nonprofit Invisible Children, which received international attention after its YouTube video "Kony 2012." The purpose of the campaign was to raise worldwide awareness of Ugandan warlord Joseph Kony's crimes against humanity and marshal the international community to take action and stop his self-styled Lord's Resistance Army (LRA) from killing and abducting numerous civilians and children. Through my involvement with this campaign, I made a friend in a native Ugandan named Patricia Akello, herself affected by the LRA violence her family suffered, who was working as an advocate for Invisible Children and whom I assisted by spreading word of the organization and of Kony's crimes. My involvement ultimately culminated when I and several other activists covered the downtown area of San Francisco near City Hall with posters of Kony, including risky methods such as placing the posters on a rotating mechanical statue and covering the nearby Orpheum Theater and its outer walls, designed in such a way to spell out "Kony" across much of the building.

By my junior year I had met a great many fellow students who were also activists looking for a common cause to rally around. That cause arrived in the middle of an environmental sustainability class I was taking where my professor, who doubled as my academic advisor, informed us that there was a rapidly growing environmental movement across college campuses called the Fossil Free Divestment campaign, where students were demanding that their universities drop investments in fossil fuel companies that were in their financial portfolios. Within hours of being told of this nationwide endeavor, I and up to twenty classmates and friends decided to start our own divestment campaign and petition the university to drop its investments in fossil fuels.

It began as a series of meetings to determine how we were to start and maintain an effective campaign with enough power to convince the university to take action on this issue. In the beginning, I was shy and withdrawn, for not only was this a new experience for me, but despite my social advances in the last couple of years, I was still self-conscious about my shortcomings as an autistic individual and was concerned about whether I was going to be an asset or a liability to this new campaign. I eventually decided to inform several of the most prominent activists in our meetings about my condition and to see whether it would hinder the plans we were making. After privately informing them, and after a couple of seconds of silence, they told me that as far as they were concerned, this was an all-inclusive cause and they did not believe I could possibly be a hindrance to their campaign, for they believed that everyone had ideas worth considering and were deserving of every chance they could get. With their stamp of approval and acceptance, I promptly began fielding ideas and strategies to help chart our mission and campaign forward. After much deliberation, we all decided that the campaign would be split into two groups, one focused on research to find information that would legitimize the need for divestment, and the other focused on outreach in order to foster as much support as possible from the student body and the faculty. As I had grown into my talent for public speaking and had a knack for persuading people to listen and ultimately support a cause, I volunteered to be a part of outreach in order to put the campaign's research to good use.

Over the course of a single semester, my friends and fellow activists, myself included, scored a series of victories in our quest to strip the campus of its investments in the fossil fuel industry. In addition to bringing in new activists, generating dozens of supporters, and looking for reasons for the board to heed our call to action, we discovered that out of approximately $80 million in the school endowment, $2.5 million was invested in fossil fuels. Through researching for precedents in our case, we discovered that divestment as a protest tactic had been used for the past thirty years, ever since protesters convinced institutions to divest their holdings in companies that were doing business with the South African Apartheid government. Historians agreed that it was an effective tactic, especially after apartheid ended when Nelson Mandela traveled to the Bay Area, specifically the University of California in Berkeley, and personally thanked the supporters of a free South Africa for helping to bring about change in his country by financially, politically, and morally bankrupting the repressive regime. Further historical research indicated that it was used successfully against tobacco companies in the 1990s, and now it was being used against fossil fuels, which made us feel assured knowing that recent history was on our side. The most important research we found was financial evidence that by divesting from fossil fuels and reinvesting in renewable energy, the university would not suffer financial blowback and could capitalize on its investments with a growing, stable, and infinite energy source with enormous monetary potential.

Bringing this to the Associated Student Leadership council and the University Affairs board quickly led to unanimous verdicts in our favor to move it up to the Foundation Board, which comprised all of the top-level officials including the university president. At the end of the semester, several friends and I attended the meeting. The board members decided that while they had a legal responsibility to handle all of their investments carefully, they had not forgotten how progressive-minded the city and community they lived in was and how the university was no exception to that. They further expressed frustration at how Ivy League schools such as Harvard were refusing to hear their staff and students and stubbornly refused to act in any way on a serious matter like this, just as they had also resisted efforts in past divestment campaigns. The decision the Foundation Board made was swift and favorable: the foundation was to immediately divest coal and tar sands from the endowments, equal to about $200,000 to $300,000, and would establish a special committee to determine how to divest the rest. As a result, my university became the first public school in the United States to divest from fossil fuels in any amount.

Leaving that meeting with my friends and activists, the feeling inside me was beyond surreal. I had never felt so happy in my entire life because for the first time, putting aside my insecurities, working with people who wholeheartedly accepted me for who I was and what I was willing to do for this campaign, and all of the enthusiasm and hard work I put into this campaign had resulted in us making history. Our professor later told us how he believed that we were the most effective group of activists in more than thirteen years. He also considered it a phenomenon that twenty people with no previous experience in this field were able to create change that was already garnering the attention of many other schools, institutions, politicians, and even celebrities. Putting this all together, I felt as if I had achieved nearly everything I wanted: something to believe in and work hard at that could lead to employment opportunities down the road, being a force behind a change that I could also put my name on, and discovering some of the best friends I could ever have asked for.

While there were still other experiences I had yet to face, such as finding a college romance, I did not think much of it for the first time in a long while. Instead of lamenting the things I did not have, I had just received most of what I had always wanted, and I was going to only count my blessings from here on out. My senior year of college was about to begin, and I was walking on air going into the final summer before I was to graduate. I already had a plan: I was going to take the divestment campaign to new heights, cement my friendships, continue to find new experiences, and most of all, enjoy my remaining time as a college student while simultaneously securing a professional job for when I finally joined the rest of the world. For me, anything was possible at this point, as I felt that my anxiety and stress was under control, my social issues were no longer feeling like issues to me, and I was beginning to feel the way I always wanted to be treated: like everyone else. The only mistake I made was thinking that it could stay this way without any more trouble on the horizon.

CHAPTER 14
CURVEBALLS AND CONUNDRUMS

It started as an unspeakable tragedy, an event that shocked everyone to their very core and beyond any belief. The image of scared children running from an elementary school as the police closed in, far too late to prevent what had occurred. I had awakened from a late night of study halfway through my junior year and was going through my regular routine of checking my social media, email, and finally the news, specifically the British Broadcasting Corporation, which I credited with giving the most impartial news of any network. Those images were the first to appear in my field of vision, even before the title registered with me: "Massacre at Sandy Hook Elementary School: 20 Children Among the Dead." It was enough to make me forget about everything that was to happen that day, enough to make me zone out in class, enough to take away my appetite, and enough for me to feel the unshakeable need to follow this story through to the end. I found myself feeling so emotional, sometimes close to tears, as I read the obituaries of everyone who lost their lives in this completely senseless act of violence—even more devastating to know that most of these lives had barely even begun—and all of the countless souls broken by their sudden departure from this earthly plane of existence.

Inevitably, my focus shifted over to the individual responsible for this, the shooter who filled a school with bullets and escaped justice by taking his own life in the process. The first thing that hit me was that his name was Adam. Soon after, what went through me like a massive electric shock was the focus taken on his mental state, which for a time, seemed to focus almost solely on the fact that he was autistic, and implied that it may have been a major trigger factor in the shooting. These reports went on for days, to the point where I was nothing short of terrified for myself, feeling that this was something that might have to be shut away once again behind my wall of denial. The difference was that I considered doing this in order to protect myself instead of convincing myself that it did not exist in the first place. For I knew all too well that there have been many points in history when something horrible happens and people want something or someone to blame, which sometimes resulted in witch hunts that led to innocent people being hurt or worse. Considering that there was, and still is, a stigma on mental illness and many Americans who have shown a propensity for violence on minorities, LGBTs, and others who act just a little bit different from their definition of a normal human being, I felt justified in how I felt, even though it invited back a heightened sense of stress and anxiety that was impossible for me to hide.

Before long, attempting to hide those feelings got the better of me, especially when I was being tutored for a chemistry class that I was struggling in and the tutors noticed that I was distant and inattentive. When asked what was going on with me, I was resistant to answer at first, but with my symptoms at unbearable levels, I confessed to them my deep-seated fear of being targeted because an individual with my name and my disorder had just committed the second worst school shooting in recorded history, with so many innocent children. My tutors then assured me that not only did they know what my disorder was, but it was also not considered a mental illness. They were certain there was so much more going on in the shooter's head than just that one issue. As it later turned out, the news reports shifted to his apparent interest in past school shootings, the many firearms present in his parents' house (*they were also gun rights advocates*), and evidence of a host of other undiagnosed mental health issues that took the focus away from his autism. With those revelations and multiple assurances from my friends, family, therapist, and people who advocated for mental health rights, I felt a degree of calm and relief finally settle over me again. My fears finally went away for good when, later on that year, I joined in the divestment campaign and its success changed my outlook.

Senior year in college finally arrived, and as I moved into an on-campus apartment in the international housing area, I already had the idea that I was going to make this the best year possible, to make up for all of the times I had never felt even half as good as I did at that moment. Soon enough, I met my roommates, who hailed from France and England, and was introduced to the rest of the international student community soon after. For the first few months, I felt like I was on the most incredible high I had ever experienced—and for the record, I did not have to smoke marijuana to feel it. Being around such sociable individuals who came from all corners of the world and who accepted me more than even the average American made me feel more sociable than I had ever felt before. From the very first outing with them, I noticed many changes all at once.

First, I was surprised by how astounded they were when it came to where I was born and how knowledgeable I was. As I learned, the average European likes to have intellectually stimulating conversations and takes compliments with style and satisfaction, as opposed to the many previous encounters I had with people (*fellow Americans*) who did not like talking at length about anything and often treated my genuine compliments with suspicion and uncertainty. Taken with the fact that I was an American who was not born in America but I had plenty of international knowledge, they took a liking to me immediately.

My second revelation was the group members themselves and the adventures they came up with. My group consisted of eight French students, two British, one Japanese, and a Mexican-American with international travel experience. Through them I was introduced to the broader international community, which often consisted of hangouts at the local bars, house parties, and late night adventures around the streets of San Francisco. It was also thanks to them that I experienced a number of firsts: my first real date with a young and beautiful Japanese student, Rie Tanaka, whom I met at a party and spent some time with before midterm exams got the better of us; my first college dance party at an Irish pub, where we all danced as crazily as if we were at a hard rock concert; and my first cultural exchange, where I invited them out to my family home in Lafayette and introduced them to California wine and the nearby reservoir. Having grown up on French wine, it was revelatory when they took the first sip, and as we walked along the pathway to the reservoir, they remarked how the weather and landscape reminded them of the South of France.

The third pleasant surprise was, and still is to this day, one of the best experiences I ever had. It was the Thanksgiving holiday and a week off from school, and Kaiser Rangel, my friend with dual Mexican-American citizenship, told us that he was planning to spend the vacation with his family on both sides of the border, in San Diego and Tijuana. Having previously worked at a fancy hotel in San Diego, he asked if we would like to come stay with him in discounted rooms with picturesque views of the city, the bay, and the naval bases. Being the jovial and all-around friendly person that he was, and because this vacation coincided with my birthday, I eagerly accepted the invitation. One eight-hour ride later, our van arrived in a sprawling seaside city I had not seen since I was a little kid, and it looked so much nicer than I remembered. Kaiser gave us the tour of the hotel he previously worked in before handing us our keys to our massive hotel suites. From there, we explored the city, going to the main park area near the zoo, Coronado Point, the sea cliffs, and finally Old Town San Diego, where we had some of the most delicious Mexican food I had had in a long time. Kaiser told us it was just a warm-up to prepare us for when we crossed the border to have a real Mexican cultural experience. It also happened to be on my birthday, which made the anticipation and the excitement exponentially greater. The morning of my twenty-second birthday my friends surprised me with a large chocolate cake and a rousing chorus of the famous French song "Champs Elysees." Afterward we drove to the border checkpoint, and following a few quick words with the Mexican border police, we were driving into a slightly more run-down city, with numerous small alleyways, street vendors, and a square full of vibrant culture with citizens and tourists alike.

The birthday celebration continued on like a dream. We ate at a restaurant overlooking the main square where I fell in love with Queso Fundido, which was essentially melted cheese with mushrooms; bought a hand-woven poncho at a flea market; stopped by the seashore where we sipped coconut water right out of the shell; and finally, went to meet Kaiser's family. His family, consisting of his stepmother, sister, grandmother, and brother-in-law, proved to be friendly, welcoming, and excited to be hosting people from so many parts of the globe. Through these interactions, I made a number of discoveries: Mexican cuisine was equal in quantity and quality, which made it impossible not to satisfy; the definition of family consisted of a large number of relatives who were close to each other, in contrast to many families I knew from back home; and there was a lot of pride in their country and identities, which in many ways rivals the pride of American identities. After getting to know them a little better, Kaiser's sister and brother-in-law took us to the downtown area, where we listened to Spanish pop music, drank lots of local cocktails, and ate plenty of food.

Little did I know, until well after the fact, that they had a surprise in store for me; they must have tipped the staff off about my birthday, because next thing I know, a whistle blew in my ear, and several waiters stuffed a large pink and white hat on my head before smashing a plate full of whipped cream into my face and forcing me to drink copious amounts of tequila. To this day, I do not know how I was able to survive the night without blacking out, but I do know how I got my revenge; it is traditional to have street tacos after tequila, so I simply "failed" to mention how hot ghost peppers were to my friends when they tried them. One friend in particular, who thought of himself as invincible, quickly rolled around in a dirty street gutter yelling about how hot it was and begging for it to stop. It was four in the morning by the time we made it back across the border to our hotel, and after an incredible Thanksgiving dinner with Kaiser and his family in San Diego, we returned to San Francisco, where in that moment, I felt like the luckiest person alive.

Underneath every picture-perfect moment, however, there often is something that has been long simmering beneath the surface, a disaster waiting to happen. The aforementioned friend who reacted badly to the ghost pepper, D.M., was one of the British students in my group who also had dual Irish citizenship. He had a background as an amateur boxer and pursued that dream until he decided to study kinesiology, which he was continuing to pursue during his year abroad. His physique was clearly defined in bodybuilding form: while not a pure muscle mass, his legs, torso, and arms had the look and feel of someone who spent most of his time lifting weights and hitting punching bags. Completing that look was a buzz cut and a face that looked like it had been beaten down by both the weather and a few fights. While D.M. did not officially live with us, he was best friends with my British roommate, and practically lived with us for the duration of the semester. At first, he was the life of the party and made the initial interactions fun whenever we went out to enjoy the nightlife and many other experiences we all had. However, as time went on, I began to realize certain things about him that were unsavory; he lived a hedonistic lifestyle, where he believed he could say and do whatever he wanted and that no morals, values, ethics, or even common sense existed in his world. While I was not against hedonism in principle, as I believe that everyone wants pleasure to outweigh pain, I did not for a moment approve of his unethical approach to the practice.

He soon began subtle attacks on my character, saying that I was a weird person beyond the standards of the city, as San Francisco has always had a reputation for being weird; he would then follow up by badgering me about my Jewish heritage, saying that because it did not come from my mother, I therefore was not Jewish, and he shoved his computer with the Orthodox principles on the screen in my face to make his point, even after I said that my Reform Jewish heritage accepted all sides. When I was not around, he would impulsively change the decor of the apartment despite the fact that the decor was my property, and in one instance, after drinking heavily, nearly destroyed my television set when he initiated a beer-spraying war with his friends. I was unsettled by his behavior, made more obvious by the fact that, after my father met him when I invited everyone to our home, he later told me his impression of D.M. was that of a thug.

Initially, I attempted to forgo any resentment of him for the sake of our group of friends, for the rest of them treated me like an equal and were a major reason why my social life had reached such heights, but also because I was afraid that if I turned on him the others would do the same to me. Tensions flared, however, when he began courting one of the French girls, C.D., a fellow dancer and a kind, fun-loving young woman with a petite physique and a radiant smile. I was unsupportive of their relationship, partially because of his burgeoning selfishness and immorality, but also because I felt the need to protect her from him. It was not out of romantic love for her; rather, I believed her to be a good person and because the dance community looks out for their own. Despite my belief that he was slowly corrupting her in his ways, as well as her increasing loyalty to him, I was able to shelve those feelings when we went on our Thanksgiving trip to the south, and was in good spirits when it was C.D. who brought in the cake and started singing "Champs Elysees" to me. The night was almost spoiled, however, when a severely drunk D.M. attempted to make a terrorist joke in front of a border patrol officer as they were inspecting our van for clearance. We were able to shut him up just in time to get through. Driving back, I hoped that this fragile harmony would last for the rest of the semester, but I ended up finding out how wrong I was in the hardest, ugliest way possible.

A week after the best birthday of my life, I was busy preparing for my upcoming finals when I heard a commotion coming from the living room. In my mind I was thinking "What did D.M. do this time?" Was he messing up my decor again? Was he making life difficult for a freshman who was rooming with his best friend, or worse, was he getting busy with C.D. on our couch again? I went into the room and saw him sitting with my English roommate and another friend watching an ultimate fighting match while taking enormous swigs off a half-gallon jug of vodka. While I went to the kitchen to get something to eat, he drunkenly called out to me to get over to him. When I approached, he shoved his laptop in my face and showed an email confirming that he would be officially moving in with me. At that point, I left the apartment, claiming I needed to take care of something, but in reality I was trying to regain my composure and figure out how to handle this news. He was toxic, there was no disputing that, for I was absolutely certain that my social shortcomings did not impede my judgment of his character. I was still trying to figure out what to say to him as I headed back to the apartment, only to discover that for the third time, he had taken down my living room decor (posters, flags, etc.) and tossed it all over the floor to be stepped on.

The dam inside me finally burst, and with it a torrent of rage came out of me. "Get out! . . . Get out of my apartment, I have had enough of this, you are not welcome here anymore!" I followed that up by asserting I would contest his admission to my apartment the next morning. Too late, I realized, I had unleashed a brazen beast inside of him that was further influenced by the many shots of vodka in his system and his reflexive boxing skills. It started as a bunch of retaliatory insults and denigrations to my integrity and character, ranging from familiar language of me being an outcast and ruining every relationship I have to curse words too vulgar to say aloud or write down. But as I held my ground, he soon got physical, gripping my left arm and smacking me in the face. The commotion soon brought in the rest of our group, including C.D., who made no attempt to stop him and tried to defend him from my assertions on his poor behavior and his need to leave. Feeling betrayed by her actions and pushed past my breaking point, I ordered them all to leave before I called the housing authority. They dragged D.M. out of the house—although he still wanted to fight—and they did not return.

It took me a few moments to catch my breath, and even longer to collect myself in order to figure out what to do next. Beneath the surface, I was shocked by my own actions, as I never wanted to start fights or make enemies, and yet here was an example of that very thing. After I reasserted myself, I immediately reported the assault to the housing authority and campus security. Although I was lightly reprimanded for my misconduct, they took my case seriously and rescinded his confirmation, banning him from freely using the building without express permission. While the campus security investigation did not officially press charges, I was satisfied knowing that during the course of the investigation, D.M. knew that I was willing to use the full force of the law if necessary.

CHAPTER 15
A CRAZY TWISTED THING CALLED LOVE

In many ways, what transpired between D.M and I ended up influencing another aspect of my personal life, one that I never saw coming, one that was slightly inappropriate, yet one I attempted to hold onto regardless of the consequences or what it ultimately became. In the initial stages of what would eventually become a mutual enmity, I initially reported my hardships with D.M. to the resident advisor, a young Asian woman named A.L., who lived two doors down from me. She was a smart, fun, and understanding person, and she was always on top of her responsibilities for the residents of the floor. She was also tall and fit, with brown hair flowing down the length of her back and a face that glowed with warmth. The first couple of times I went to talk with her, it was about my problems with D.M. and some of the insecurities I had about finishing up my senior year of college.

There was a subtle hint, however, that I picked up on in those encounters; even when our business was concluded, the conversation kept going. It was rare for this to happen to me with anyone, which is why I found it peculiar. The third time I went to see her, she moved the meeting to her room and locked the door, ostensibly so we would not be interrupted. While I spoke to her, I noticed how close she was sitting, how she was at rapt attention to every word I said, and most of all, the glow in her brown eyes as she stared at me without blinking. It was then that I noted that there may be something there with her, and I also began to notice something there with me too. There were several more encounters, both official and unofficial, where we were dancing around the unspoken attraction between us, mostly through distracting small talk and the continued issues I was facing. At the same time, I began to learn a lot about her history: She was the daughter of Cambodian refugees who lost their parents in the genocide perpetrated by Pol Pot's communist regime, and she grew up in Orange County before moving to San Francisco to attend my school. In addition to her background, she was also a Buddhist and had recently switched her major from business administration to political science. By the time I told her how I felt, she returned those feelings to me, though she asked that we take it slow for the moment.

When I returned from my trip to San Diego and Tijuana, the first thing I did was visit A.L. and tell her how it all went. By the end of my story I told her a secret no one knew: when I made a wish in front of the birthday cake my friends had given me, I wished for the impossible. My birthday did not mean as much to me as I wanted because she was not there with me. While I am not the kind of person who betrays personal interactions and intimacy to the general public, what I will say is that what came next was too good to be true, because up until that moment nothing like that had ever happened to me before. It was perhaps due to this encounter I became so enamored with her that I wanted to spend more time together. Several days later, she asked me to come to her room again, only this time, I detected a more serious tone in her voice. We sat down and she pointedly asked me what I wanted with her. Because it has never been in my nature to lie, especially about the most important things, I told her that because this kind of thing never happened to me before and was everything I ever dreamed of, I wanted to be with her and to be someone who she could always count on to support, cherish, and above all, grow to love and mature with together. I also acknowledged how questionable it would look in the eyes of the housing authority if they knew she was with someone she was in charge of, which is why I was willing to keep it quiet until the end of the year when there was no need to hide anymore. Despite my declarations and my willingness to compromise in certain ways, she asserted that she could not lie about a relationship for that long a time, that she had been hurt in two previous relationships by men who promised their hearts to her, and that she was uncertain if it would work long-term because of me leaving school before her and with other things she planned to do on her own. At the time we mutually agreed to take a break and keep some distance between us, but that did last long.

After the massive fight I had with D.M., A.L. was the first person I reported the assault to, and she passed it on to the housing authority, which subsequently led to his ban from my apartment. Within only a few days, however, she went back on her own assertion and invited me back to her apartment for another intimate encounter, which resulted in us continuing to spend time together, culminating in a kiss under the fireworks by the ferry building during the New Year's celebrations and a fun night out drinking at a nearby German gastropub. As quickly as it happened, however, she went back to the same boundaries as before. Being who I was, I was confused and upset by the back-and-forth nature of our connection, and I could not stomach being strung along like this. I finally sat down with her and confronted her about the state of our relationship, to which she replied that while she certainly felt and retained the same feelings as before, she could not bring herself to confirm them for the reasons we had discussed previously. She went on to say that it could not happen between us, at least not right then and there, and while she did see a future for us, it would not be anytime soon.

In hindsight, it was a test she was giving me, a chance to "man up" and accept the situation while still keeping her in my life as a friend, to which there may have been a chance for us in the not too distant future. Instead, socially and romantically inexperienced as I was, I allowed for all of my memories of social abandonment and all of my personal fears to take hold, and over the course of my final year, did whatever I could to keep her close and convince her that I was worth being the man she would want, that she was the first person I could imagine having a real future with, and every beautiful thing that came with it. Inevitably, I did the wrong thing for the right reasons, and the supreme irony of it was that I ended up pushing her away, to the point where it has been years since we last saw and spoke to one another. That blunder of mine is one I still consider to be one of the most emotionally devastating blows I have ever endured, for I was inspired by how my parents met in college and made it work so many decades later. I realized far too late that had I done what she asked, she and I would most likely still be in each other's lives at the very least. When graduation came and passed, I reluctantly accepted that what was done had been done and it was time to move on.

INTERLUDE II
IMPRESSIONS AND THE LITTLE THINGS

"In youth we learn; in age we understand." — Marie Von Ebner-Eschenbach

Going through those transformative years in college reminds me of the aforementioned *tabula rasa* and how we are continuously defined by what we experience and the state of the environment that we grew up in. The experiences and the environment I spent four solid years in did indeed bring with them events that left lasting impressions on me, many of them going into the present day. One of the most important lessons I learned during my schooling came after reading about spirituality: the teachings of Tibetan Buddhism, and in particular, the teachings of its leader, the Dalai Lama. He preached that the true enemies in life were the feelings of anger and aggression, which meant that if there was someone you hated, that hate alone made you as bad as that person was to you.

As such, he believed that only kindness, compassion, and happiness were what are necessary to achieve a peaceful, fulfilling life. As a result, I began teaching myself meditation and practicing the simplest forms of Buddhism, in which I never harmed a living thing, allowed for my anger and aggression to be replaced by passiveness and understanding, and most of all, attempted to have these feelings supersede my stress and anxiety. The last of these practices produced mixed results, but nonetheless gave me a measure of control over my emotions.

I also discovered sensitivity to certain substances that others did not find inhibiting. For example, I have only ever had two hangovers in my entire life. The first came after a night of heavy drinking with my international friends. I meant to have only a single shot and a pint of beer, but before I knew it, they were pouring several shots down my throat along with several more beers. I was on the verge of blacking out, so I somehow managed to haul myself back home where I experienced all of the negative effects that came with excessive drinking and the subsequent hangover. To be in such a state of pain left a strong impression on me. My friends and other experienced drinkers constantly preached that the more hangovers you had and endured, the more of a man you would become, but instead, it made me never want to experience that again. My second hangover would be years later due to underestimating the power of mixed drinks, but luckily, I did not go through the worst of the symptoms.

Slowly, I have learned to appreciate the little things in my life. My dog and my two cats have been a major part of my life for over a decade, but I did not always see them that way. Because of how consuming my anxiety and self-consciousness were, I often put my angst and drama before their concerns, which led to my parents being their primary caretakers. This went on for all of high school, but while studying in college, I was exposed to numerous instances of the effects of animal cruelty and negligence through the testimonies of animal rights activists, haunting images, and graphic videos. These encounters shocked me into realizing how I had taken for granted my own pets for so long. From that point on, whenever I came home from school and into the present day, I did everything I could to make up for lost time and take as good care of them as possible. In the process, I also discovered the importance of pet therapy. While it may be true that pets do not understand what you are saying, the fact that they still listen and do not say mean things back to me released many emotional weights off of my back. It felt good just knowing that there was a living, nonjudgmental animal by my side to make me feel happy again. In turn, I wanted to make them feel happy and well-cared for, which is why I have now taken pleasure feeding, walking, and caring for them.

When I would walk my dog, I also began taking stock of the natural scene around me, the vast, green expanse of woodland and fields that surrounded the town, reminding me of how simple yet beautiful the flora, fauna, and distant hills were in those moments. Simply hearing birds sing and seeing their natural habitat not only reminded me what I was fighting for as an environmentalist but also brought about a sense of peace and calm that fit right into the Buddhist teachings I was learning. Even in San Francisco itself, the parklands and protected spaces in and out of the city offered me that same sense of peace and made me feel like there was not a single worry for me to be concerned with. However, just as an appreciation of the little things can give me a sense of peace and happiness, so too it can have the opposite effect. These little things, effectively, can be placed on their own spectrum of good and bad, with the scales tipping back and forth depending on the situation. Many of the problems I have faced throughout my life did not always come from big events; rather, as the saying goes, "The devil is in the details."

Focusing on problems that, in hindsight and to others, did not seem like major issues still felt exactly like that to me; it was easy to pour so much stress and anxiety into them. Whether it was an upcoming college exam or attempting to accept circumstances in my social life, the associated feelings would amplify the issue much more than it needed to be, which often made problem-solving feel like one impossible situation after another, often leaving me in a state of indecisiveness over what to do.

The one thing I have been able to take comfort in throughout my four years in college was that compared with the previous four years, the good far outweighed the bad. If not for having the freedom to forge my own path, the variety of areas of study open for me to pursue, and the many kind, mature, and understanding souls I met along the way, my time in college would have been no different than what happened before. The first two years involved some adjusting and figuring out who I was and where I fit in, but by the time I reached the latter half of my college experience, they were without any doubt in my mind, the best years of my life thus far. My junior year began that special and impactful journey for me, and senior year capitalized on it. To say that my graduation came with a broken relationship and the loss of some people I called my friends to sum up the experience would be quite inaccurate, for during that time, a number of truly wonderful events took hold and made me fully believe in myself once again.

CHAPTER 16
HOPES, DREAMS, AND HIGH NOTES

It could have been the end for me once again, a major fight resulting in the loss of many friends who, just a week ago, gave me the best birthday celebration of my life, further aggravated by the unraveling of my relationship with A.L., all on the cusp of my final semester of college. But that was what the younger and more inexperienced version of myself would have thought and accepted as fact. The truth could not have been further from that perspective, for all of the advancements I had made throughout the last few years were coming back to show me that I still had so many other things to cherish and look forward to.

Fresh from our historic victory in convincing San Francisco State to divest itself of the dirtiest of fossil fuels, our campaign began to push on to greater heights than ever. Although we lost some of our friends and fellow campaigners to graduation, we made up for it with new recruits and greater ambitions, the latter of which involved keeping the pressure on the school to deliver on further divestment from the remaining fossil fuel money in the endowment while simultaneously transforming our campaign into one that spanned the other twenty-two college campuses in the state university system. During this time, two phenomenal things happened to me on a personal level in relation to my work with the campaign, both happening at a Halloween party several weeks before my trip to Mexico. The first occurred while I was watching my friends winning a game of beer pong in the apartment garage. I was approached by a young woman whom I did not realize was female as first because of how she was dressed up in an immaculate costume of the rapper Lil Wayne (*She was not of African descent and definitely not wearing blackface, but had the dreadlocks wig, hip-hop clothing style, and fake tattoos all in the exact imitation of the man himself*). She gave her name as Emma Hedermo, an international student from Sweden, who was studying behavioral psychology during her year abroad. At first, I was nervous to talk with her, believing that I would be boring, but when I told her about my involvement in the divestment campaign, it was as if a fire had ignited within her eyes. The next thing I knew, she was pressing me for details, telling me that she was looking to get involved in something bigger than herself and that this sounded like the perfect opportunity to aid in a cause that society and the environment depended on. In the months following, Emma, as her blonde, blue-eyed, bohemian musician self, not only became an integral part of our campaign, but she was also responsible for connecting us with like-minded activists in her native Sweden and other places outside of the United States.

The second amazing incident of the night occurred shortly after my initial conversation with Emma. I had moved to the second floor of the apartment where the rest of the Halloween party was in full swing. It was here that I ran into a familiar face: Kate Hallett, a red-haired, slightly bookish-looking British student who had visited us during the first campaign meeting of the semester. As we talked, she told me that she was only in San Francisco for a single semester and was not convinced that she had enough time to properly aid in our efforts. I encouraged her, upon her return to England, to start a campaign at her university and continue the fight there, as I had learned that many campaigns were beginning to form across the world. Having not thought too much about it from that point on, I was taken by complete surprise when I received an email from Kate months later telling me that she had assisted in the formation of her university's divestment campaign and how they were already close to getting their foundation to divest from fossil fuels. She ended her email saying "thank you for inspiring this movement." I nearly broke down in tears of joy, for I had never imagined up until that moment that a casual conversation I had at a party would lead to one of the greatest moments ever to happen to me and the campaign, and it only went up from there.

My involvement in the divestment movement exposed me to what felt like an entire ecosystem of activists in the environmental social justice field, and with it came new opportunities and new friends, one of whom became one of the best friends I could ever ask for. It began when Marli Diestel, a fellow campaign founder, and I were hanging out at a bar with friends from both my international group and the campaign. She was about two-thirds my height, with long red hair, a kind, pale face with a nostril-piercing, and a clothing style that looked like a cross between throwback hippie and modern bohemian. Having been at the end of yet another one of D.M.'s drunken taunts, I was outside getting some fresh air and collecting my thoughts when Marli came out to see how I was. As I let her in on my insecurities and shortcomings as a social individual, she told me something I did not expect in the slightest: that whenever she spoke to her family in her hometown of Chico (*the same town as A.K.*) and they asked her about people she studied and worked alongside with, she would tell them that the person that worked with her, gave everything to his studies and a cause, and was an overall kind and inspirational human being, was me. I was a person she looked up to and who she believed knew what it meant to be devoted to something bigger than oneself, while being inclusive of everyone. Thanks to that unexpected act of kindness, our friendship cemented and we continued moving forward together.

Through Marli, I met many other people who became allies to our cause, including several in the student government who granted us an audience with student representatives from every state university in the California system. For the first time, I was to be the one to speak on behalf of the campaign to convince them to adopt a resolution that would guarantee support to other divestment campaigns from every student government in the system. While it was initially nerve-wracking, I reminded myself of the success I had the first time I spoke during my final presentation for my hip-hop workshop several years back, and I subsequently approached it in the same way, taking care to be as informative and articulate as possible, letting my voice sound like it had command of the subject, being persuasive yet receptive of all opinions, and being prepared to answer any questions. By the time the meeting ended, over a dozen student delegates approached me and said that the campaign could not have chosen a better person to relay the message and encourage swift, decisive action in favor of a university system free of the influence of fossil fuels, to which they pledged serious consideration and, in some cases, support.

Success followed success as a network that spanned the country and spread into Europe began to take form, with our campaign being a major part of the expansion and bringing in more people and supporters with every passing day. My role continued to grow, and before I knew it, I was attending city government meetings and forums, communicating with activists through conference calls, and even being one of the organizers of a major gathering of activists across the country dubbed the Fossil Free Convergence. During that time two things happened that cemented my abilities as an activist and a public speaker. The first occurred when I successfully convinced a city supervisor to join a panel of officials scheduled to take questions at the convergence regarding their views on divestment and how it influences politics and policy. The second came when the other organizers granted my request to be the opening speaker for the convergence, which would require me to give a rousing speech to over three hundred people from all corners of the nation. In what was arguably one of the most nerve-wracking yet successful moments of my life, I gave a speech in which I encouraged everyone present to show that our millennial generation has the power to shape the very fabric of society to protect the environment and allow for nature and society to peacefully coexist for generations to come. Seeing them all stand up for me, cheering in unison, and later congratulating me for kicking off the convergence in the greatest way gave me a sense of inner peace for the first time in my life. I finally felt like I did not have to hide any part of myself, that I was now just like everyone else, normal and accepted. In that moment, the wall had finally collapsed into oblivion.

The rest of the semester continued like a dream; even after the fight I had with D.M., while I did indeed lose the group of friends I had spent time with because they were always with him and did not condemn him for his actions, there were many other international students who defended me, including Emma, who was appalled by his behavior. Another Swedish student, Dennis Greunlund, the captain of the school hockey team with the athletic physique and long shaggy blond hair and beard to go with it, even offered to teach him a painful lesson. I turned him down, but through that act of solidarity we became good friends. I continued to make other friends, inviting a Dutch classmate of mine out for drinks, spending time in Golden Gate Park with my fellow environmentalists, hiking Twin Peaks, and fully immersing myself in San Francisco life. Eventually, I traveled with many friends and fellow activists to Santa Barbara for a sustainability convergence, where my circle of friends grew. I also went to nearby San Marcos to make a final plea to the student representatives of the state university system to vote in favor of a system-wide divestment campaign support, which passed with a comfortable majority.

As the semester was coming to a close, and with it my college experience, I took time to reflect on everything I had gone through and came to the conclusion that I had finally achieved just about everything I wanted out of life: here I was, half a lifetime later, surrounded by true friends, having overcome incredible odds to prove myself on the social, political, environmental, and academic track, experiencing mutual attraction and the beginnings of love for the first time—all things that only a few years before I did not believe for a moment I would ever have the chance to experience and hold on to. In addition, I had finally accepted myself as an autistic individual, found ways to reasonably manage my stress and anxiety, and even with my differences from the average person, still managed to be myself and be a part of an inclusive environment where I was as normal as the definition of the word. These reflections and feelings followed me as I prepared for graduation, putting on my cap and gown, being fitted for a college ring, and being confirmed as a cum laude graduate—having been on the honors list for all but one semester—and for my dedicated service to the university. Seeing my parents and extended family at graduation and their looks of pride and admiration further validated my feelings of accomplishment and self-worth, and they gave me the strength to give a speech to my graduating class. I spoke from the heart, showing my admiration for growing up beside them and espousing my belief that we were all part of an extended family bonded not by blood, but by the fundamental belief that society and the environment could and would coexist peacefully because we were the ultimate solution to the problems of the present and future.

In the week following graduation, I celebrated with my family and friends, including spending an extended afternoon and evening with Emma, whom I had grown to greatly admire as an activist and as one of the most humble, vulnerable, and above all, beautiful human beings inside and out. When she left to get ready to go back to Sweden and already having to accept that many of my friends were going to leave San Francisco for pastures anew, I felt a sudden upheaval of emotion, for it was beginning to hit me just how hard it was to say goodbye to the greatest chapter of my life thus far. I shed a tear as her bus slowly disappeared into the busy evening traffic. Emma represented one of several tiers of friendship to me; she was the friend I made through my activism and my social interactions with foreigners. The other friendship tiers were those of whom I was friends with through classes, through roommates, and through the many random chances that blossomed into recurring interactions and ultimately lasting connections. While these friendships had varying degrees of connection and presence in each other's lives, I treated them all as equally important to me, hoping that they all felt the same and would keep our relationships strong beyond our days of studying and adventures. Even with the end of an important chapter of my life, I reminded myself of all I had accomplished. I had practically run a massive campaign, worked alongside nonprofits in support of it, grew and developed into a socially relatable person, graduated with honors, and above all, had my whole life ahead of me. In my mind, I had already achieved the impossible, I knew exactly what I wanted to do with my life, and so now all I had to do was go to work. After all, with everything I had accomplished, who could possibly say no to me?

STAGE THREE
ADULTHOOD

"Try not to become a man of success, but rather try to become a man of value" — Albert Einstein

CHAPTER 17
CRASHING FROM THE HIGH

In this modern age, the generational shift among millennials has been an obvious one: where there was once a time where college graduates would immediately find employment and a place to live to begin their independent lives, most of them now face a stark reality where they have to rejoin the families they left behind four years before. My case was no exception. Immediately after graduation I was back in my Lafayette home, back in the town I swore I would move far away from, back into my room on the third floor, with its moon-shaped window facing the valley and town, with my shelf/desk hybrid in one corner and my loft taking up another and built into the wall seven feet off the ground. Having a place to sleep and plenty to eat made it easier to accept, but with the deep sense of accomplishment I still felt and a strong sense of confidence coursing through my system, I was certain that in no time at all, I would be landing a meaningful job like my parents did and putting my career into high gear. On my computer was a list of between twenty and thirty jobs I was ready to apply for. Some of them were directly involved in supporting the divestment campaign, which I believed would be the reason I would find employment so quickly, having built those connections over the last several years. Furthermore, with my field being part of an ever-expanding section of the overall job market, I was even more confident that employers would want plenty of eager young job seekers fresh out of college to join in that expansion and the many responsibilities there were to advance the green economy and the overall civil sector (*nonprofits, campaigns, foundations, etc.*) that was already drawing in so many.

My descent was gradual yet full of punishing blows. While I had expected some rejection from certain jobs, I never once stopped to consider the possibility of each and every single one of my job choices rejecting me in steady succession. I attempted to convince them in every way I could think of: a polished resume; the many references I had from my previous campaign and internships; a session with a career counselor to make the best, most professional cover letter; and even going as far as, for some jobs, acknowledging that I had a disability if it meant giving me an advantage in hiring, though I stressed that it had never limited me in my ability to work in any task I was given. Despite my best efforts, every single job I applied for turned me down, whether it was a polite rejection email or no communication at all. Having to make an entirely new list of possible jobs was excruciatingly difficult, as I did not have many other options outside of the organizations and the movements I had been a part of. Other sectors, while similar in scope, the required experience and skills were beyond my own. The weeks turned into months, and before long I had regressed into my reclusive habits. Trying to fill the hole drilled into me by the rejections, and to calm my mind, I binged on television, movies, and video games, having no friends left in the town. While I managed to get outside a decent amount of time to walk my dog and visit my friends who remained in San Francisco, it was no longer with the same feeling of making every moment in my life count.

My enthusiasm and commitment to a cause greater than my own was slowly slipping away from me because the cause was not there for me when I needed it the most. Nonetheless, I continued the fight as best as I could, flying to New York four months after graduation to participate in the People's Climate March on the United Nations that brought nearly half a million people marching through the streets of Manhattan. In addition, I joined an intercollege organization called the California Student Sustainability Coalition to stay connected with the people I had worked with, in addition to staying up to date with the movement and providing as much assistance as possible. Unfortunately, because I was back in a town that brought back troubling memories, I wasn't in college anymore, and I had to accept that many of my friends were not planning to make San Francisco their home after graduation, I could not bring myself to find the same joy and commitment that had fueled me for years, nor could I separate it from the feeling of needing my passion to be linked to necessity. In other words, any attempt to keep my enthusiasm and interest in environmental social justice required me to have a financial incentive, and because education was no longer a part of it, it had to be part of whatever kind of employment I could attain.

The more I searched for work, the more my stress and anxiety levels continued to climb. Beyond the apparent futility of my efforts was also the prevailing question that, as time went on and I did not put what I learned in school to good use, would there come a point where I have been inactive for so long that my skills and knowledge would become obsolete? My parents continued to urge me to search widely and not go a day without applying for a single job, convinced that tireless work and dedication would eventually result in a successful hiring. Despite their urging and support, I could not help but wonder if after all this time, they still did not see that the endless applications with zero acceptances was eating away at my self-esteem , that the job market had significantly changed since they were my age, and that putting pressure on me to continue the same way only resulted in amplifying my bad habits and reactions to failure.

I had applied to the Peace Corps, believing that working abroad would reinvigorate my desire to do good and be productive while also giving me a new perspective in another part of the globe. Upon being accepted and receiving my assignment, I discovered that I was going to the African country of Zambia, where I would be on my own, living in a mud hut, an hour's bike ride away from the nearest Peace Corps member, and needing to learn any one of a dozen local languages in order to communicate with the local populace and be productive in my work, all during a period of twenty-seven months.

The sweat began to form, my heart started racing, my breathing barely able to remain steady as I zoned out while reading the acceptance letter. There was no excitement or optimism in any part of my mind, only stress, anxiety, and sheer terror at the thought of living by myself in a rural countryside with no security, having no real sort of income, and being forced to learn a local dialect when I had already failed to learn Spanish after several years of study. Nothing I did could calm me down, not thinking about it more positively, not meditating on it, nor taking several days to sleep on it. Eventually, I decided it was not worth it and turned it down, though not without a lot of regret over the only job to accept me at that point. Luckily, my parents comforted me, saying that they actually would have been surprised if I had taken that position without hesitation. There was nothing more for me to do except to move on with my job search, so the journey continued.

After weeks of sporadic activity on the job front, I decided to look at programs in AmeriCorps, the domestic equivalent of the Peace Corps. Having traveled many places in my life, I had not spent much time exploring the country of my citizenship. AmeriCorps would also give me a chance to help many Americans who needed assistance, as poverty rates were substantial, environmental issues were prominent, and volunteering for a federal government agency would bring a lot of experience and skills to my resume and set me up for looking better on paper for future jobs. With that in mind, I began applying to AmeriCorps, ultimately finding eight programs, including a few environmental options, in and out of California that I believed I could handle if given the chance. All too soon, seven of those programs turned me down, and I was back to believing that this was another waste of time. That was when the final program came through for me, a hybrid program called FEMA Corps, which combined traditional community service with working directly for the Federal Emergency Management Agency. It was a ten-month program in which I would be a part of a team of volunteers in my age range traveling the United States working with many disadvantaged communities and the various regional branches of FEMA. With no other options to pursue, and with encouragement from my family, I accepted the position and waited for the initial instructions to arrive.

It did not take long for the forms and the informational packet to show up in my inbox, and all too quickly, a familiar feeling crept back into my psyche as I attempted to read the volumes of requirements and steps to prepare for the ten months of service. Despite attempting to look at this in a positive light, a combination of an overwhelming amount of information and a general fear of the unknown incapacitated me with the worst amount of stress and anxiety I had ever felt. It was like having a nervous breakdown; I could not properly control my breathing, it felt like there were weights pressing in on my chest, and no matter how much I willed myself to fight it, there was no stopping it, for it lasted the entire time I forced myself to read everything and did not leave until I had removed myself from in front of my laptop screen.

My parents tried to convince me that everyone in my position felt this way at the start of something new, whether they were looking forward to it or not, and that as long as I followed the rules and kept myself as busy as possible, everything would work out in the end. Furthermore, they encouraged me to embrace it as an adventure, since I had been on many of those before, including when I flew solo for the first time to New York for the People's Climate March.

A familiar experience I had hoped not to go through again with someone so close to me was one factor in my eventual decision. After that incredibly fun party I had invited him to years back, S.S. and I were in regular communication, until one day he inexplicably ceased all contact with me. For two years I did not hear anything at all, and no one else who knew him seemed to have any answers either. Then one day he returned to Lafayette. He told me that he had been in and out of school, had dealt with a difficult breakup with a long-time girlfriend, and had just felt at the time that it was best he did not involve anyone in his issues as he tried to figure them out for himself. He apologized to me and said that he had left Southern California and was trying to put his life back together again while attending school in Berkeley. Naturally, considering the ten years of friendship we shared, I forgave him and rekindled our friendship with the promise of remaining close. As the time to depart for FEMA Corps training neared, I asked him to spend one more day with me in San Francisco, in order to enjoy the time we had left. He readily agreed and we made a plan to meet at the train station at noon the next day. When morning arrived, I called him to make sure we were still on for our planned rendezvous; there was no response. I nonetheless went to the station at noon to see if he was still showing up. An hour later, there was still no sign of him. I never heard from S.S. ever again.

It felt like it was the breakup of my friendship with Z.M. all over again, the only difference was that the former gave convoluted and possibly coerced reasons for ending things while the latter just vanished without a word. The pain was just as incapacitating as before, and I found myself wondering why the last of my friends from Lafayette had just up and abandoned me right when it seemed like we had reconciled? No matter how hard I wracked my brain to understand what had just transpired, I could not comprehend what the cause of all this was. Was it me? Was it him? Did he figure out my autism, become scared, and thought of me as a hopeless burden? Had something happened that I did not know about that he felt he could not share with me? Was someone whispering in his ear about me? All of these theories swept through my mind, but with no evidence, no indication of why he did it, and with no one to provide any kind of answers for me, I felt hopelessly alone and friendless for the time leading up to my federal service.

While I still felt some reluctance, I nonetheless resolved to break personal barriers and feel more independent from my parents while embracing a new adventure in my post college life. The ulterior motive was to try and numb the pain of my lost friendship with S.S. and hopefully create stronger, lasting friendships going forward. I would spend the next three weeks preparing for my service through basic training in Sacramento, which would be on the grounds of a former Air Force base. There was some comfort in that, knowing that my maternal grandfather served more than twenty-five years in the Air Force, that my uncle had served in the Marines, and that now, even though it was not the military, I was about to go and serve my country in a different, yet nonetheless helpful and significant way. When my green, army-style travel bag arrived and everything was packed away, the day arrived to ship out for training. My parents and I hauled everything into the car and began the ninety-minute drive up to McClellan Air Force Base. For once, my parents were both acting calm and Zen, perfectly in sync with each other, assuring me as much as possible that while this new experience felt daunting, I would adapt and do some incredible things as part of a team of volunteers for America. Deep down, I hoped that this would also be an experience that would rejuvenate my spirit and add to my skill set for future employment opportunities.

CHAPTER 18
STICKS AND STONES WITH SMOKE AND MIRRORS

From the first day of training we were awakened at four in the morning over the course of the three weeks to undergo intense physical training, alongside team-building exercises. We were put into the teams we would be with for the duration of our service. We had come, all 130 of us, from all corners of the country to serve as "Volunteers for America," and we would be treated and cared for as such, or so we were led to believe. One thing that was made clear was that we had to follow the rules of the Corps or we would not be allowed to continue in the service. This seemed simple enough to me, but not so to others, resulting in a number of people being cut during training because of actions ranging from insubordination to underage drinking among younger volunteers. Even with the training, the cuts, and the barrage of different exercises, duties, and curfews we endured, my reluctance was slowly ebbing away, as I was beginning to believe that this would give me the purpose I desired, and I was reminded that this would help me give back to my country.

I was part of an eight-member team, comprising three men and five women. Like every other team, we were under the direct supervision of a team leader, in our case, a young woman named J.T., a graduate student from North Carolina. She was a short, stout young woman with a blonde bob and glasses covering a pale and slightly heavy-looking face. She came off as a sweet, understanding, yet grounded and committed individual who wanted us to be the best, most efficient team we could possibly be. She kept her promise of making us into her vision of a team as we diligently handled our duties and often volunteered for more, as we kept up with our physical training regimen and determined what our individual roles would be and how they would complement each other. She was so convincing in her demeanor that I decided, in the interest of team unity and there being no secrets between us, to inform her of my autism. Her eyes flashed in a kindly fashion as she graciously thanked me for my honesty and promised to accommodate me as best as she could. Before long, other team leaders began giving us praise as the most well-behaved, efficient, and in-sync team on the base, as many were complaining of disciplinary issues and losing some of their team members who had decided to go home.

The only drawback for me during this period was that I had to be certified to drive a van that our team would use to travel the country. Despite having years of practice and owning a driver's license for the past five years, I was still a reluctant driver. I had always felt an elevated sense of anxiety and alarm whenever I was in the driver's seat, whereas in the passenger's seat, I was as Zen as a Buddhist monk. Despite expressing my misgivings as a driver, J.T. assured me that I was one of several drivers she would need so I would not have to deal with being behind the wheel all of the time, adding that she was certain I would get used to it over time. It certainly did not feel that way as I went through the certification test, my hands gripping the wheel like a squeeze toy, droplets of sweat appearing on my forehead, and the fear of something unexpected around the corner coming too fast for me to do anything about. Even after I passed the test, I felt no more confident than I did when I first hauled myself into the driver's seat of the large ten-passenger van. As we approached the end of our basic training, one of our teammates received the news that she was to be transferred out to a specially designed unit that would be working at FEMA headquarters in Washington, DC, for the entire year of service. That brought us down to seven members as we left Sacramento and headed to San Luis Obispo for a week of FEMA training on a National Guard base.

The next round of training proved more difficult, as it involved understanding special government computer programs that were far outside of my comfort zone. Having to be in a classroom with a number of other volunteers who did not seem too bothered by working on these programs brought out the worst of my self-consciousness, as I felt like I was the person who was asking for help more than the rest of the class combined. I had heard all of the generalizations and stereotypes on autistic people being smart when it came to computers and the science and programs behind them, but that had never been me. These programs were more foreign than any language I had seen or heard of, and my lack of comprehension came out in my agitation, cold sweats, and constant seeking of assistance. Thankfully, with the help I got I was able to push myself through the training, and by the time we were ready to ship out to our first destination, I was looking forward to the work ahead of me, believing that once we had arrived, I would not have to worry so much. We were informed that our ten-month service would involve three project rounds in which we were to be in different places in the United States, assisting with whatever was needed.

For our first project round, our newly designated task force was assigned to Texas, specifically the town of Denton, just north of Dallas. For the first three days we drove across the Southwest, traveling through Arizona, New Mexico, and finally through Northern Texas on our way down to Dallas. Initially, it was fun and exciting, seeing the desert regions for the first time while traveling along the famous Route 66, watching the scrublands elevate into sheer canyons and valleys full of wildlife, along with rustic houses of Native American design scattered around enormous plots of land. Every now and then a city like Albuquerque would emerge from the desert like a mirage, and we would be back in civilization again to stay the night before venturing on in the morning. Entering Texas opened my eyes to a lot of flat prairies and ranchland along with animals like the burrowing prairie dog rodents and various birds of prey circling the holes above. By the time we reached Denton and the surrounding towns, we were exhausted yet curious about our new surroundings, which consisted of many different parcels of flat land, some with commercial properties, some residential, and the rest fields and forests, all scattered around as far as our eyes could see. Having finally arrived, my team and I were eager to begin our service as soon as we possibly could.

The veil fell away from the very moment we arrived at our lodging. The FEMA Corps system quickly proved to be one in which we would receive information at the last minute, and it was never good news. We were told that we would be living in a Lutheran Bible camp in the middle of a parcel of woodland in a number of ramshackle cabins, cut off from the rest of the Texas populace. It quickly became apparent that these cabins were not the safest places to live in, as some of my teammates discovered scorpions, mosquitoes, snakes and other dangerous, invasive animals in our cabins, along with a lack of adequate plumbing and questionable electrical power. Having another team temporarily living with us did not help matters as we were barely able to find enough space for ourselves. After a difficult first night, another call came in for us: contrary to everything they told us before, and made even worse that almost no other teams were being affected by this, we were ordered to remain in Texas for the duration of our service. Being robbed of our chance to see and serve the entire country infuriated many of us, especially me, as I was already beginning to suffer from a number of maladies. I had long suffered from spring pollen allergies, and while I was often able to control them, the pollen was so powerful and widespread in Texas that my medication had no effect at all. On any given day I felt like I was suffocating, with an itchy throat that felt like it was covered in hives, along with streaming eyes and a runny nose that made it difficult for me to concentrate.

Despite these unexpected setbacks, I persevered along with my team to look past our decrepit conditions and focus on the work we came here to do. Most of that work would consist of us working directly for the FEMA regional headquarters that covered several southern states, as well as doing community service for local organizations whenever we could. The FEMA facility we worked in was unlike anything I had ever seen: it was a Cold War–era bunker with several floors underground, with offices, meeting rooms, and a command center. Our office space was right next to the command center with dozens of government computers, a screen with live weather patterns, and a number of manuals and other official books on emergency response and recovery. In addition to the bunker, there were some above-ground buildings where logistics and training personnel worked. My first two weeks on the job was in one of those buildings, where I worked on inventory, counting the compound supplies with one of the federal workers, a humorous, light-hearted African American man named Kelvin, who originally hailed from Chicago. He showed me every inch of the facility as we catalogued various items (*walkie talkies, computers, FEMA guidebooks, etc.*) and introduced me to his colleagues. It was thanks to him that I began to enjoy the practical and social aspects of my service, despite the issues my team and I were having with the program itself. Because of his kindness, fun-loving personality, and patience with explaining the ins and outs of the base, it was Kelvin who helped me grow into my role and become more accustomed to how federal procedures worked around there.

Within the first couple of weeks, there were some stark contrasts about our situation. Although I was enjoying the work I was given, the FEMA Corps program itself was, in many ways, a lie. They had convinced us that we were these specially chosen volunteers for service to our country who would be accommodated as long as we were dedicated to our work. But in reality, we were a cheap, expendable labor force with few rights and even fewer services to assist in our needs and issues. Decisions on living conditions were arbitrary; there were few people to talk to about our issues, as there were only two program therapists with limited time to speak with and understand us, and individual concerns sent up the chain of command would either go unanswered or be swiftly dismissed. To the program brass, we were only as good to them as the service we provided; it was we either dealt with the way the program was designed or leave altogether. As a result, every week there would be news about Corps members leaving the program, and while there was some initial action taken to deal with our living situations— moving out of our cabins to an extended stay motel closer to Dallas— it only lasted a month before we were sent back to the same camp, albeit with slightly better accommodations with little animal infestation.

To add further insult to injury, it quickly became apparent that J.T. was not the same person I knew from training camp. Despite informing her of my condition and how an unfamiliar environment brought out the worst of my anxiety and stress, when it subsequently occurred, she took it personally, to the point where she would force me to face difficult issues in a way that felt abusive. It began with subtle insults like negatively comparing my ability to concentrate, comprehend information, and achieve results to my teammates and FEMA personnel. It soon moved on to criticism of how I looked and presented myself in the workplace, such as if my uniform was not perfectly creased and straightened, and not to ask questions or make statements she believed were impertinent. Furthermore, she expressed disbelief at my inability to fully comprehend instructions and computer programs that the rest of my team picked up without much difficulty. Being autistic, I had some difficulty with multi-step instructions, both before and during this program, and the anxiety from that continually disrupted my concentration and made it impossible for me to memorize specific details of such instructions and programs. But that did not seem to make any difference to her. I tried to think critically at first, wondering if maybe I was overreacting to the entire situation. Perhaps I was unintentionally causing trouble for her because she was our team leader and under a lot of stress managing us. When I privately brought this up to my teammates, they unanimously assured me that I was not crazy, that while they had also been exposed to her unscrupulous behavior, it was nothing compared with what she had been doing to me from the start of our project round.

The reality of how she was treating me began to sink in. Despite my best attempts to reconcile with her to preserve team unity, I repeatedly failed to mend fences between us, and her callousness continued unabated. She found fault with my interest in other government projects, such as wanting to do assignments for the Environmental Preservation and Native American Tribal Affairs sectors of FEMA, when she believed I should simply be following orders and doing whatever she assigned me. She also refused to comply with certain dietary requests I made when we were shopping for the team, which resulted in me dealing with severe stomach cramps when forced to eat certain foods that did not mesh with my digestive system. I had to give up drinking coffee when the brands she had us drink artificially induced stress and anxiety when there was no reason for me to feel it, which made for terrible mornings when I arrived at the bunker (*To this day, American brands cause those symptoms, while foreign blends have never done this to me, possibly due to a lack of synthetic chemical additives found in American products*). While diet may not seem to have anything to do with being autistic, the fact is my condition already influenced how I viscerally reacted to stressful events, and J.T. forcing me into uncomfortable eating and drinking habits only compounded the same symptoms and their effects. Despite all of these stressors and clashes, I refused to quit or let it stop me from doing my job, which often led to more positive encounters with the federal staff and opportunities to get to know people and the surrounding southern US landscape better. Examples included assisting in emergency drills with the Dallas police department, updating contact information of the personnel in satellite offices in the region, and even organizing regional staff meetings with officials from around the country, including the director of FEMA himself.

Near the end of our initial project, our first major emergency occurred. The command center became filled with dozens of federal staff, security, and military officials running point on different stations in response to a series of tornadoes that had hit Oklahoma and northern Texas. It was so intense that we sometimes spent up to thirteen hours at a time working in the bunker. It was during one of those times that I was working alongside one of the civilian response officials electronically tracking resources being sent to the disaster zones to aid with recovery efforts and the survivors who needed assistance. During a break he asked me what I thought of my service in the FEMA Corps. Being that it was not (*and still isn't*) in my nature to lie and not always knowing in the moment what the right thing to say was in a given situation, I told him that while the program was not what I expected it to be, I nonetheless was proud to serve my country and assist the government in giving the aid and assistance so many people desperately needed from us. He seemed satisfied with my answer, but J.T., who was sitting nearby, was flabbergasted, as she mistakenly believed she heard me airing personal grievances and openly criticizing FEMA Corps and by extension, FEMA itself. As such, she dragged me out of the command center like a naughty kindergartner and demanded to know why I would say such horrible things to a government official. I fired back at her, telling her that was not at all what I said to him and that I was through with her assuming the worst of everything that came out of my mouth. It quickly devolved into an argument about my autism where, finally pushed to my limits on how callous and apathetic she was to my condition, for the first time I fully defended myself as an autistic individual, telling her that there is no changing how I am developmentally wired and that she needed to accept who I am and deal with any social shortcomings and ineptitudes that come with it.

 I have stated before how I have good memory recall, but it is often not good enough to recall full conversations I had with people in the past, but in this case, it is impossible to forget the next words that came out of J.T. 's mouth. Her exact words were as follows: " It looks like we've reached an impasse.... If this really is who you are, then I don't see how I can possibly help you anymore, and coming from my experience in the professional job world, I cannot think of a single employer who would ever want to hire you based on who you are and what you just said to me." Because I was in a defensive posture, physically and mentally, the full impact of those words did not sink in until after we got back to the campground. It was as if she had put a vice around my ankles, attached them to hundred pound weights and threw me into a river to drown.

After all the times that I had attempted to fix things between us, to make things better for the team and put the needs of our country ahead of our own, here she was, unrepentant in her behavior, set in her convictions, and making comments that were borderline bigoted. It was not long before my other teammates began to feel the same weight of her attitude, and several of them made plans to leave as soon as they possibly could. While I can never be sure, the fact that they had their own issues with J.T., that they already acknowledged how she disproportionately focused her aggression and negative energy on me, and that they had the ability to extricate themselves from her influence and FEMA Corps, gave me the impression that nonautistic individuals could solve complicated social situations and create multiple contingency plans the way I could not. Sure enough, by the time we returned to Sacramento for our debriefing and a short summer vacation to follow, one of the girls in my team left for home, planning to join a local work program in order to get away from AmeriCorps. As someone who could not conceive a viable path out of the program and who felt trapped as a result, I envied her for being able to leave, especially with what came next.

In the beginning of the program, I became close to a young woman named Ariel Tyson. A native of Tampa, Florida, African American with sweeping brown hair and eyes that flashed with excitement and energy, she was part of a team that was going to spend its first project round in Washington, DC. From the very start, I was able to bond with her in a way that I was hardly able to with other women. She laughed at all my jokes and other quips about her sassy attitude and habits, we had serious talks about real world issues where we always found common ground, and we were both fascinated with each other's backgrounds and stories. Throughout the first project round, we stayed in close touch, often having video chats on our phones and updating each other about our respective adventures.

By the time we came back to our base, I was relieved to finally see her again, but that relief would not last long. It soon came to my attention that she was being accused of stealing a personal item from one of her teammates. The item was never found in her possession nor anywhere else, yet her accuser was standing by her statement. I fully expected the unit leaders to dismiss the issue because it was just a "she said, she said" situation; instead they arbitrarily expelled her. My faith in the program was shattered when I found out, made worse when J.T. stood by the decision, saying that the unit leaders knew what they were doing and that the decision was for the best. Seething with anger, I decided to rebel against the system and started by intercepting Ariel as she was being taken to the airport to be sent home. While I did not physically meet her there, I contacted her by phone and convinced her not to board her flight. Instead, I offered her a chance to enjoy what little summer break we had and turn it into a worthwhile adventure, and I had just the right plan to accomplish that.

CHAPTER 19
A BRIEF RESPITE AND A RETURN TO MADNESS

It was Mother's Day, a few weeks earlier, a month before the project round was to end. My team and I were relaxing in the campground, enjoying the day off we had from the bunker. I separated myself from the group to call my parents and wish my mom a happy Mother's Day. Instead, they had a surprise of their own for me: they were selling the house I had lived in for twelve years and moving to a smaller apartment in San Francisco. While I had always hoped that we would one day put our life in Lafayette behind us, I nonetheless was shocked that they were choosing now, of all times, to do so when I was so far away and slated to stay away for a long time. In my mind I was wondering what would happen to all of my possessions, how they would be handled and not be lost. Also, because I was attached to a lot of our other family possessions, what would happen if my parents sold off something that I wanted because it had been with us for most of our lives? Despite these concerns, it turned out to be a blessing in disguise, especially when Ariel and I arrived at the house, now empty of our possessions but staged for sale while my parents had already moved into the new apartment.

Knowing that we had gone behind the FEMA leadership's backs, sidestepping their attempt to send her home and having a great vacation ahead of us gave me a sense of glee I had not felt since college, when I was fighting for divestment from fossil fuels. I had been part of something that was all about fighting the current system. Now I was again. As such, I was going to make sure that I gave Ariel the best vacation she could have asked for. It all started with taking her to several different restaurants around the Bay Area, given that she was a prominent "foodie" and obsessed with rating her experiences online. Then came the usual sightseeing adventures in my city, from the twisting shape of Lombard Street to the Irish coffees at the world-famous Buena Vista cafe. Those were soon followed up by visits with my family in the new apartment, which had great views of the Bay, and shopping around Union Square where Ariel introduced me to a homemade cosmetics shop with items I would consider buying for my mother for her next birthday. During that time, it became apparent that we had feelings for each other, and because our time together was limited, we had to make that time count.

As stated earlier in this narrative, I do not betray the more intimate details of my encounters. But from my perspective as an autistic individual, there were many things that happened that were too good to be true, as the more neurotypical individuals experience these things with less difficulty almost to the point of routine. In a way, what happened between us was a lesson in what was possible. I had to treasure every moment I had, so I went out of my way to make her feel special and like she was the luckiest person in the world. When the time finally came for her to return home, we promised that we would always be there for each other, that our future significant others would simply have to understand. As such, we parted on emotional yet very good terms.

As soon as our vacation ended, so too did all of the good vibes that came with it, as I rejoined my team with J.T. as stern and unapproachable as ever. I also caught up on news from the other teams, only to find out so many people had left the service that some teams were disbanded with their team leaders bound to the base to work off their service in administrative roles. This discovery convinced me even more that I was not alone in the belief that this program was fundamentally flawed, but unlike those who left, I was not someone who quit so easily. Because I had already endured four months of service, along with certain things I did enjoy about being in Texas, I knew I had to see this through, and I resolved to continue working and looking for new opportunities. Sure enough, when we arrived back in Texas, my professional and personal life improved ever so slightly. I spent time with my teammates enjoying the Southern hospitality Dallas and the surrounding areas had to offer, going to different bars, playing laser tag and bowling at the nearby arcade, and going to the state fair and trying all of the fried foods the South was so famous for. I did not, however, enjoy them as much when J.T. joined us, for even outside of work, she was annoying, had irritating habits, and often felt more like an intruder than an actual part of the team. As the weeks went by, several more members of my team left the program, until there were only four of us left. While I was always tempted to do the same, I had to constantly remind myself that this was bigger than me and I needed to stick it out. A lot of this determination came from being reminded that while I was still in high school my parents gave me the chance to transfer schools to try and escape my torment from my classmates; I had steadfastly refused because I would never allow myself or anyone else to believe that I was a coward who ran away from his problems.

On the work side, I was catching the attention of some high-level people. The chief of FEMA operations for our region, a fit, middle-aged African American man with a serious, weather-beaten face who liked to be called "Bullett," a name he had gotten from his years serving in the military, began taking an interest in my eagerness to help with certain projects. Having seen my work and assistance with certain tasks like updating government contact information and organizing staff meetings, he gave me an assignment I could not refuse. Because I had worked with the facility's tribal affairs liaison on assisting Native American tribal governments, of which there were many in Texas and Oklahoma, he asked me to do something that no one in FEMA Region VI had ever done before: create a section on tribal governments for a FEMA strategy guide used by officials and leaders like him. It needed to provide as much information as possible on the many tribes and to suggest ways to assist them and improve cooperation between FEMA and the tribal authorities whenever they are affected by natural disasters. I quickly realized how significant this was; he could have asked any salaried federal employee to do this, yet he was entrusting it to an on-loan volunteer like me, and I knew that I could not let him down. Despite my ever-present anxiety and my concerns about how J.T. would react knowing I had gone over her head for this, I dived into my role, tracking down all information I could get from the FEMA servers I had access to and coordinating with the Tribal Affairs office to find updated facts and reports. I wanted to build a framework for a section that would outline how to get the two sides to collaborate despite centuries of mistrust between the tribes and the federal government. Bullett gave me a month to complete the project, and because of my dedication, focus, and personal interest in the project and having studied Native American culture in college from time to time, I ended up creating a complete and comprehensive tribal guide in just two weeks, to his surprise and satisfaction. As a reward, he wrote me a letter of recommendation for future employment and graduate school opportunities.

Near the end of our second project round, I had come back from work to the Extended Stay motel we had stayed in during our last project round. J.T. was gone for the weekend and the team and I finally had the place to ourselves. The first thing I did was turn my laptop on and check email to see what I had missed while I was working my usual eight hours in the bunker. There was only one new message from my father, so I opened it to see what he sent me . . . and my soul split in two. In several paragraphs, he detailed how several weeks ago, my mother had gone to her usual doctor appointment and had come out with a diagnosis of breast cancer. The rest of the letter attempted to assure me that there was nothing to worry about right away, that they were starting treatment immediately, and that I should continue on with my service as usual. Those words meant nothing to me; my anxiety was through the roof and I was already pacing the room, my mind imagining the worst, the gears spinning like they were in freefall, my hands gripping my face so hard I almost cut myself in several places.

Once I had regained some of my composure, I knew the only true assurance I could get was directly from my parents, so I contacted them through my phone's video chat. Seeing them helped calm me down a little more, and seeing my mom still looking like her normal self—with her full head of blonde hair, her practically ageless skin, and her sweet confident smile—brought added comfort. The first thing they said to me was to not leave the program for them, as they were confident that they could handle what came next and would only contact me if things were not going the way they hoped. With a heavy heart, I reluctantly agreed and attempted to continue on with my work.

Depression was the one thing I could not put aside, and while I was able to continue with my work and broaden our volunteer efforts by working at the Dallas Zoo and painting the house of a FEMA employee, it was impossible for me to put my concerns about my mother behind. One day, several weeks after we started our third and final project round, I decided that I was going to use the few days of leave I had racked up during the year to go home and check on her. I went to inform Bullett, whom I was still doing assignments for, about what was going on and how I would have to step away from my responsibilities for a little while. To my surprise, the usually no-nonsense operations director showed great sympathy for me, telling me that the exact same thing had happened to his mother, that she survived, and that he believed for me to keep my head in my work I needed to be there for her, so that when I came back, I would be more assured of the situation and be ready to work with renewed focus.

The weight of the depression that had been keeping me down lifted ever so slightly as I returned from work to the Bible camp, where, to my chagrin, we were sent back to once again for our final project round. At this point there were six weeks left in my service and despite how close it was to the end, I was relieved to be looking forward to a short break from the usual routines and being back in San Francisco again.

The van pulled into the campground and as we approached the main cabin, J.T. stepped out of it and ordered us inside. She had been absent from the bunker that day, claiming to have both personal and program business to take care of. We went inside and sat across from her. Bluntly, and in no uncertain terms, she told us that we were reassigned to South Carolina, where there were massive floods and a lot of survivors that needed our help, and that because of the urgency, we were leaving the next morning. She finished by turning to me and saying "Your leave has been canceled."

The temperature suddenly felt like it had climbed twenty degrees. My vision was fading into a blurry image as my blood pumped at a ferocious speed and what felt like a beast was rising up inside of me. All that was in my mind was the belief that she had stolen the time off that I had earned, for me and my mother, who was only just beginning to deal with the unpleasant side effects of chemotherapy. I also felt the need to make her pay for what she just did to me. Whatever rational part of my mind that remained knew what had to be done before it was too late, so instead of raging and storming at her, and possibly doing something more that I would much regret, I raced out of the main cabin and toward my own, my mind suddenly feeling like it was no longer a part of my body. My vision continued to be hazy; I could only vaguely see what I was doing. By the time I reasserted myself, I was sitting on the porch of my cabin, my legs drawn up to my chest, with lawn chairs thrown all around the front of the cabin, a dime-sized hole in one of the walls where I had apparently kicked my foot. I retreated into the cabin and called my father to inform him of what had happened, and he told me to talk to the higher-ups to see if anything could be done. I then spoke with my unit leader, whom I had already gotten to know and who was aware of the difficult time I was having in the program. Having lost her father to cancer a while back, she sympathized with my situation and approved of five days' worth of leave for me to see my family before I had to fly to South Carolina.

Upon arrival in San Francisco, I was beyond relieved to be home again and was desperate to see my family and help in any way I could. Seeing my mother again was a blessing, especially since, despite having been through three rounds of chemotherapy, she still looked more or less the same. I caught them all up on what I had been doing in FEMA Corps and subsequently began planning how I was going to help them while I was here. I had unwittingly timed my arrival perfectly for what was to come.

The night after I arrived home, my mother suddenly developed a high fever, and before long was gasping, wailing, and writhing in pain. Although I maintained a mostly stoic face, inside I was being torn apart, for there is nothing worse than seeing the ones you love the most having to deal with such extreme pain and wondering if they are going to come out of it. My father, after conversing with doctors on the phone, promptly took her to the emergency room and told me to take care of the apartment, our dog, and two cats until I heard back from him. For three days, I stayed home, scared out of my mind over what was happening at the hospital and what I should do about AmeriCorps in light of this emergency. Finally, my father returned home and told me that in addition to her cancer, she suffered a bad reaction to the chemotherapy, which resulted in the ravaging of some of her internal organs, mainly her gallbladder and liver. It further emerged that they had not told me the entire truth: I had been led to believe that they were doing standard chemotherapy before trying an experimental trial, but in reality they had done it the opposite way. Out of about five hundred people involved in the trial, my mother was one of only three people with the kind of side effects she was currently suffering.

I visited the hospital the next day to see how she was doing. Walking into that hospital was, and still is to this very day, one of the hardest things I have ever done, made even harder by the state she was in when I finally laid eyes on her. In many ways, it is extremely difficult to bring myself to describe what I saw, though I will go as far as saying that because of her liver damage, she was suffering from severe jaundice. Upon seeing this and the pain she was still in, I came to one conclusion without hesitation: there was no going back to the FEMA Corps for me. If I boarded my flight for South Carolina and something worse happened to my mother, there is no way in any kind of universe that I would ever have been able to forgive myself.

I told my father of my decision and went about contacting both the program therapist and my unit leader to inform them of my intention to leave the program. Once again, my unit leader sympathized with me, telling me that she would have done the same thing in my position. She added that despite my early withdrawal, I was still going to receive a number of commendations for my service, including an education grant for future schooling and two medals of service from both Congress and the president because I had exceeded expectations for the number of hours I worked throughout my term.

After getting off the phone, walking into the living room, seeing the broad expanse of the San Francisco Bay and the surrounding cityscape from the floor to ceiling windows of my parents' living room, smelling the cool, slightly salty breeze, and hearing the foghorn in the distance, I knew without a doubt that I had done the right thing and that I would not miss being in FEMA Corps for an instant. Nor would I regret leaving when I did. At the same time, I also needed to acknowledge that my departure came at a major price: beyond my mother's illness, I also had to deal with my own inner turmoil, for all of those days of stress, anxiety, depression, and seemingly righteous anger had taken such a toll that I had come close to turning into something I had never been before. That something was a cold, unfeeling individual who nearly lost control in a public fashion to the point where I did not feel like I was connected to my inner self anymore. Where I once thought that my symptoms were things I had no choice but to live with, I now believed that there was something else that could be done. Just as my parents needed my help now, so did I with myself, and I was finally going to get the help I needed.

INTERLUDE III
RESPONSIBILITY, REGRET AND ACCEPTANCE

So many times, so many places, so many people, and so many regrets. And I was only twenty-four. People say that life is too short to be filled with regrets. I have seen and felt the effects of certain people's actions, when they say or do something and express no regret or remorse afterward. These actions have often occurred where any sensible person would feel ashamed and regretful of what they have said and done. It often begs the question, are we actually ignoring things we should regret and just taking responsibility for them to convince ourselves that we do not have regret in our lives? Does that make our lives better or feel like it lasts longer? Is it that bad or that hard to feel regret, feel remorse, and then accept it and move on?

The truth is we all make mistakes (including me), sometimes big ones, sometimes hurtful ones. For every stumble I made—from attempting to make friends with someone who had a problem with loyalty, to falling in love with someone whom I should have been more mature with, and finally, almost succumbing to pure animal instinct when I had a knee-jerk reaction to attack J.T., who delivered the message that almost kept me from my cancer-stricken mother—I always felt the deepest feelings of remorse and regret for what I did when I came to my senses. In my mind, lying was impossible, was a sin, and in some cases, made me physically sick. Therefore, I never had an issue taking responsibility for my actions, to myself and to others. Knowing just how close I came to losing control of myself in both my mind and body the day before I left on my reinstated leave, feeling the physical strain my stress and anxiety had on me, and experiencing the mental anguish from my depression finally convinced me to seek more intensive help. My belief at this point was that I badly needed to atone for my actions and find a way to give penance, even if it meant finding a more aggressive solution such as psychiatric attention.

Because of those feelings, along with needing to be my best self while taking care of my mother, I made an appointment with a psychiatrist at the University of California, San Francisco, hospital in order to see if I needed to be checked in for treatment. Talking to her, I found that it was not difficult for me to describe things in detail, good or bad, easy or difficult, right or wrong. Perhaps it was my belief that lies make things worse; that ignoring, covering, and omitting important details does not help me in any way; and moreover, burying pain, loss, and feelings only leads to further suffering and eventual self-destruction. I managed to give her a nutshell version of my life story, detailing my initial diagnosis of autism and how the various symptoms that came with it influenced my life. Furthermore, I explained how recent events had compelled me to find a deeper, more permanent solution, if there was any to be found. After listening intently to me for a couple of sessions, she commented on how I was good at describing my symptoms in such detail. In addition, she did not believe that my condition nor my actions warranted being checked in for inpatient treatment at a facility. She offered me the chance to be a part of a short outpatient program in which she would carefully evaluate me over the course of several more sessions. By the time those sessions had ended, around six weeks, she prescribed to me an antianxiety medication known as citalopram. She said that it would be able to tame the anxiety and depression I felt with great effect, though she warned me that relief would not be instantaneous. Within three days of taking it, it was as if a thick, suffocating veil had been lifted from my body, the veil being the constant air bubble in my chest, the rapid beating of the heart, the shaking in my legs when I tried to sleep, and the constant concern over the little things that felt much bigger. I no longer felt depression for every other thing that was wrong in my life, and I could finally talk to my parents about serious topics without getting into anxiety-induced arguments with them.

The best thing about getting the medication was not the effect it had on my system and demeanor, but rather the relief of knowing that taking responsibility for myself through seeking help brought me to this moment of self-improvement. By seeing that I could manage my symptoms and allow for the best parts of me to appear in my everyday life, I could be more accepting of myself at all levels. While it was, and still is, by no means a cure-all for me, it did allow for growth in my social life and my personal development. I accept the parts of me that were not, and still are not, perfect. The major lesson learned from this—almost ten years in the making at this point—is that I will be able to learn and develop my way out of certain issues that held me back on a social and mental development level. But I also learned that there are areas that will never change that I have to accept as imperfections to live with. One of those imperfections that not many people have but that I fully believe to be true about me is that when I attempt to drive a car anywhere, my anxiety and stress overwhelms me and I react viscerally, and my medication apparently has no effect. That situation, plus some research I did, brought me to the conclusion that I have what is called vehophobia, or a literal fear of driving. Despite all of my attempts to get used to it over the years, I have had to accept that this was something that is never going to change, so I gave up driving shortly after this realization and have not been in the driver's seat in the years since. That decision was, and still is, one of the few I have never regretted, especially as an environmentalist, because I believe there should be fewer cars on the streets anyway.

Overall, the cycles of regret, taking responsibility, and accepting myself for who I am, while a long time coming, were well worth it in the end. While it is true that cycles themselves never end, I believed that going through them with a willingness to better myself and making lasting improvements to my life would make the process more bearable going forward. As I settled back into my life in San Francisco while planning to take care of my mother and find another job, I made another decision. Simply put, while erring on the side of caution in certain situations, I now fully accepted that I was an autistic individual. I still see myself as normal in many ways, but I also accept the ways that I am not, such as my eccentric mannerisms, my need to be more self-aware, and my working harder to nonverbally read people better. Most of all, I see myself as someone who only ever wants to do the right thing for myself and everyone else in my life, to help others however I can, and to be happy. The wall of denial is truly no more.

"That person who helps others simply because it should or must be done, and because it is the right thing to do, is indeed without a doubt, a real superhero." — Stan Lee

CHAPTER 20
LEARNING TO BREATHE AGAIN

It was a tricky balancing act: bringing my mother home, while also trying to honor her wishes to find employment and keep myself busy, on staying on top of the therapy sessions I was attending. When starting to look for a job in my field once more, I went in with more confidence than I did last time, for I had made a good impression in my FEMA Corps work that, despite my early withdrawal, resulted in a letter of recommendation from my former FEMA supervisor, newly arrived medals and commendations from Congress and then-President Obama, and a more extensive skill set on my resume and online job account. Despite not officially graduating from the program (*I later found out only 53 out of the original 130, including my remaining three teammates, made it to the end*), I convinced myself that I had a better chance than before. Those first six weeks proved me wrong all over again. I applied to more than a dozen jobs, including a number of city government jobs I thought were good bets to hire me because of my work at the federal level, only to have none of them to give me an interview. With the realization that nothing had changed, I reluctantly searched for work in the local area so I could at least save as much money as I could.

Going back to basics seemed to be the logical step for me. While looking at what movies were playing at our neighborhood theater, my mother told me she had seen job openings at the Sundance Cinema in nearby Japantown. Being close by, having a great set of mainstream and independent films, and offering a much larger minimum wage than I had ever earned at my high school theater job made for the best possible position for me to apply to. Soon enough, I was hired and back in a new, yet familiar landscape. There were significant differences, however: the staff was much friendlier and accommodating, not all about business and profit, and my coworkers were more into their work and treated each other like family, which made for a more pleasant experience and something to look forward to with each shift. With my mother's condition going up and down, I felt obligated to inform management, and they turned out to be understanding and sympathetic and balance between work and being available for her. Over time, I made friends in the workplace, many of whom indicated that I was a funny, friendly, kind, and understanding person. Some of those descriptions were familiar, others not, such as being funny and outgoing, for I have many memories of being quite serious and humorless. I remember how jealous I used to feel watching my gregarious father casually humor and charm everyone he ever met, never believing I could be capable of the same, and now here I was, doing a similar thing with my friends, colleagues, and, occasionally, customers.

Having now become accustomed to my medication, I had a much more optimistic outlook on life once again, and I felt that my hard work, friendly relationships, and commitment to my family was beginning to make up for the erratic and borderline dangerous behavior I had previously been guilty of. When it came to caring for my mother, I was there to encourage her when she was not feeling strong mentally and physically to keep giving it the good fight, along with taking care of things she normally did but did not have the strength to do so, mostly cleaning the apartment and placing potted plants (*tulips and ferns were her favorite*) around the living room and kitchen. I also tried to ease the burden on my father, her main caregiver, who was beginning to show signs of stress and weariness as my mother's fragile state took its toll on him. I would take care of my mother's two cats and Dash, our cattle dog/border collie mix; do chores for him; and occasionally take him out of the house to do fun things to get his mind off his difficult routines for a while.

Over time, I managed to balance both my family and my work commitments without causing too much strain on me. I began earning money, saving the vast majority of it for the future, and soon became involved in activities outside of the house. A prime example is when Greg Gee, one of my colleagues, encouraged me to join his gym, and from then on our time was spent working out together and having adventures around the city, like running around Crissy Field and trying out the best Korean barbecue in San Francisco. During those excursions I also learned a lot more about him: he was from a Chinese-American family that had lived in San Francisco for centuries, since the Angel Island immigration years of the twentieth century, and was dedicated to his Christian faith and acts of charity. In addition to his friendship, it was going well at work too. I was able to effectively manage my responsibilities and still bond with upper management, for example when we talked about Bay Area sports or the hype behind the upcoming sequel trilogy of Star Wars. Apart from still being tacitly guarded about my autism, I did not let it hold me back any longer, as I did not stumble in my speech, say the wrong things, and felt confident I was finally able to be funny.

It was not, of course, all sunshine and rainbows, for like anyone, I continued to make mistakes here and there. One time, when serving as an ID security guard for the bar inside the cinema, I took someone's word that they were over twenty-one. Even though she was of legal drinking age, I was not authorized to make such arbitrary decisions, and I was temporarily demoted to usher staff until I worked my way back to my original position. In addition, I was also forced to make a difficult decision regarding my opportunities for graduate school. I had been admitted to the Middlebury Institute of International Studies, a prestigious school in nearby Monterey that offered me a scholarship for a master's degree in international environmental policy. There was just one major drawback: even with the scholarship and an educational grant from FEMA, along with my savings, and even after I deferred for a year to earn more money from my job, it got me no closer to covering the total tuition/living expense price tag that went well into six figures. My parents urged me to take out student loans and said they could probably assist me in paying them back once their current medical bills let up. But I refused to consider being heavily indebted, so I reluctantly withdrew from enrolling in the program. As a fiscal conservative (*practical reasons, not ideological*), I strongly believed that racking up debt through student loans would take years, if not decades, to pay off. My attempts at researching other graduate programs in the surrounding states resulted in the same conclusion: any school would render me penniless long before I obtained a master's degree. Feeling a sense of defeat, I put it all aside and continued to save money and occasionally looked to see if other, more professional work was out there for me.

I came close at one point, when I was granted an interview for an environmental education position with San Francisco's Department of the Environment. I spent the better part of a week preparing for the interview, putting together a short presentation, figuring out whether to go in business-casual or business-formal clothes, and reading up on what to expect in both the interview and the job, even going as far as acting it out with my father. When the day arrived, I did everything that I believed to be right, from my presentation to answering their questions as satisfactorily as I possibly could. They asked me to check back in a week for an answer, but when I did, they told me I did not make the cut and someone else had better qualifications. My first professional interview in two years, and I had failed again. With a heavy heart weighing me down like one of the barbells I used at the gym, I went back to the usual routines of my theater job. The job with the city, which is an expensive one to live in, would have made it easier for me to afford to move out of my family home once my mother was healthy again. Having something to do— the theater job and helping my parents—cushioned the blow of failure from that interview and allowed me to continue my search for something better. Even then, I still had to contend with certain nagging thoughts about why almost nothing in the professional job process had changed for me. Were these employers on to me about my disorder? Was I a target of disability discrimination? My parents and I had read some articles about such actions that denied disabled people opportunities and reinforced chronic unemployment and/or underemployment. And why, despite keeping busy and adding even more job experience to my resume, was I still being treated as if I had not accumulated this experience at all?

Reality certainly had a way of being unfair and unkind, but it did not come anywhere close to matching the events that occurred during that time at home. Eight months after I left FEMA Corps, my mother had surgery to remove her tumor, was pronounced cancer-free, and was told she only had a 10–15 percent chance of recurrence. While she would continue to have even worse problems with her liver, this was nonetheless a major victory and lifted all of our spirits. I had known so many people who had lost the battle with cancer, including the same type that my mother had just overcome. This news completely validated my decision to leave my service in AmeriCorps; I did not regret it for an instant but most certainly would have if I had not come back for her when I did. Even though the overall battle was not over yet, it brought an unspeakable happiness to my father and me that greatly lightened the burden we had been feeling for so long. So, I began to focus on myself again, and I returned to something I had known about for a while but had never taken the time to consider: the Birthright Israel program. In my final year of college, at the suggestion of a friend, I had begun attending weekly Shabbat (*Jewish Sabbath*) at a Jewish community house known as Hillel, the largest Jewish campus organization in the world, where I made new friends and learned more about the Jewish community and my heritage. It was there that I learned about Birthright, and now that my mother was steadily on the mend, it was time for me to focus on myself a little more.

The Birthright program was special because it was almost completely free: all you had to do was go through the interview process, confirm your Jewish heritage (*in my case, through my father*), and pay a refundable deposit before being assigned to a traveling group. Whatever I spent would be on souvenirs and extra food outside of what they gave us. Before long I was on a flight that spanned half the globe as I made my way to Tel Aviv. The trip itself was life-changing, as I had never been to the Middle East before.

Knowing only of the dangers of the region constantly portrayed in the media, I was not prepared for the beautiful, unspoiled landscape with thousands of years of history preserved so perfectly you could feel its presence everywhere you went. Because the program lasted only ten days, I did not have enough time to truly appreciate it the way I wanted to. Still, the most important lessons I took away from it were the rich cultures surrounding Israeli Jews, their commitment to honoring thousands of years of traditions, the simple yet significant cultures of nomadic Arab Bedouin tribes, and the overall sense that despite the centuries of conflict that have continued into the present day, there was a good chance that this Jewish nation and the surrounding territories were closer to achieving peace than ever before. Perhaps the best lesson for me, personally, was getting to know the forty-plus people who joined me for the trip. They came from all corners of the United States, with a couple of them from other countries. They also had many different backgrounds—some in the tech industry, others with encyclopedic knowledge of pop culture, and even more who were sports and bodybuilding enthusiasts. Despite all of this, there were two important things that tied us together: we were united in embracing our Jewish culture, and we wanted to bond on a deeper level than how we would in our home countries. I discovered the latter while we were camping in the Negev, a desert region in Southern Israel.

It was at the tail end of a massive dance party in a Bedouin camp that was hosting many Birthright groups in addition to ours. We had gathered around the campfire by our giant tent: the forty of us participants, our two counselors, our Birthright guide, and seven local Israelis serving in the Israel Defense Forces, as is required for every man and woman who graduates from high school. I am not entirely sure what made me do it, but while warming up by the fire, I started to make a speech. I pointed out how the name tags we were wearing around our necks that identified us as Birthright participants were pink in color, and because of that, it held a personal meaning to me. I then told them about my mother's fight with breast cancer. After telling them that she was cancer-free, I asked them if I could sing a song. I have almost never sung in public due to the ridicule I went through in school and because I am more of a dancer than a singer, but there was something about being with them that made me want to do something outside of my comfort zone, and to sing a song that meant a lot to me while I was away in FEMA Corps. I subsequently sang "Home" by Michael Bublé, which, to my great surprise and windfall of emotion, I received a massive round of applause and cheers from everyone.

Immediately following, an incredible and unexpected thing happened: several people, group members and Israelis alike, began telling their own vulnerable stories that they would normally find extremely difficult to tell anyone about. As the one that inspired them to do so, I am honor-bound to keep their stories within the campfire circle in which they told them, but what I can say was that I went in telling a personal story without ever expecting it to have the ripple effect that resulted. Several of my group members later told me that I was a major reason that we all came together the way we did by the end of the program. I had not felt as validated as I did just then since I was in college, and the feeling is something that goes beyond any word to describe it. For the rest of the trip, I was close to just about everyone in the group, whether it was joining them for parties in downtown Jerusalem, walking through the Yad Vashem Holocaust Memorial, or showing gratitude to each other near the end of the trip as we gazed down at the Tel Aviv skyline from the Jaffa lookout point.

Coming home after giving some long and rather emotional good-byes, I felt something I had not experienced in several years: I could breathe again. My mother was through a major part of her health crisis, I had become close to a number of same-aged peers I had only known for two weeks, and I had a job in which I was making decent money and was socially accepted by everyone, from the ushers all the way to the top of the management chain. Even more, I had fully embraced myself as a high-functioning autistic individual with decent social skills and a minimal amount of medication to manage the anxiety and stress that were the worst of my symptoms. While I still had yet to find employment in my career field, I felt happier and more confident coming home, for I had found acceptance half a world away for who I was and believed that some way, somehow, it was going to happen here in San Francisco or somewhere in the surrounding Bay Area soon enough. I would definitely like to think that the experience in Israel was transformative enough that I came back a changed person, one that I was happy to embrace.

CHAPTER 21
ONE DOOR CLOSES

The battle was over, but the war was yet to be won: for a full year my mother continued to deal with the permanent state of damage her liver was in. The permanence was made clear to us several months after I returned from Israel. She and my father were told that the only way out of her liver disease was a liver transplant. The only good news was that the hospital offered to cover the expenses of the procedure. She was also told that she would go straight to the top of the liver transplant waiting list, which was organized by blood type, and being AB+, her blood type was rare. For eight months we waited for an available transplant, during which we made contingency plans for potential living donors within the family, including me. The doctors told me, after a series of tests, that I had the most compatible liver, which made me the primary candidate for the procedure. Discovering that, however, filled me with dread. Despite the rapid recovery process and how my liver, after removing the large section to be donated to my mother, would grow back quickly, there would be permanent scars and I would have to be careful for the rest of my life with certain things that most young people would never have to worry about otherwise. As a result, a familiar feeling crept back into my life: that sense of complete and utter indecisiveness, often the product of my stress and anxiety. Throughout my life, this feeling would occur with even the most trivial of choices and in circumstances like picking out a treat from many options, but in this case it was about whether I would volunteer to save my mother's life. The feeling of being in an impossible situation weighed heavily on me, for I believed there was a potentially major cost to my well-being if I went through with it. Because of my indecisiveness the hospital board decided to drop me as a potential donor, while assuring me that they had other options almost as good as me.

The decision brought an onslaught of guilt and regret. I pictured my mother's face . . . so crestfallen and disbelieving at the news, the revelation that her own son, who sacrificed so much to come home and take care of her, was unwilling to commit to giving her the part of a healthy liver she might need to live the rest of her natural life. At the same time, both of my parents had said repeatedly they didn't want to go the living donor route because of the burden it placed on other people. They much preferred, they said, to find a donor another way. But the months were mounting with no word from the hospital, my mother's eyes and skin were still yellow from jaundice, her skin intolerably itchy, and she was hearing stories about the number of people who die on the transplant waiting list, waiting for a call that never comes.

In many ways, the guilt felt so much worse than my concerns about being the one to give part of my liver and have limitations and possible consequences for the rest of my life. This kind of guilt was one that swallowed me up like a flood, and where I was drowning slowly in the consequences of my inaction. It even made me question that, were I not socially inept and besieged by high stress and anxiety, would I not have hesitated from the very start? Would it have been no question that any sacrifice was worth it for my family, that my condition was proving in this moment that I was a weak, insecure, and hopeless hypocrite?

After several weeks of struggling with the board's decision to release me from consideration, I came to the realization that I had never considered myself to be, nor had I ever been, a coward. I decided I was going to contact the board and demand that they take me back into consideration. Before I could inform my parents of my decision, however, we began to receive calls from the hospital about livers that had just become available. The first two calls turned into dead ends; one went to an individual more ill than my mother, and the other one became unavailable after the family withdrew consent for organ donation, even after my mother had been told to show up at the hospital for surgery the next day. These calls left her increasingly dispirited with the process, having already had to deal with liver dysfunction for over two years. However, a week after she began receiving these two calls, a third one brought us the news that there was a liver ready for her and that no one else would take precedence. She had to get to the hospital right away for the procedure to begin.

They left for the hospital at the same time I had to report for work, and they told me to keep up the usual appearances until they could give me news on how the procedure went. As it turned out, the doctors did not begin the operation until late at night, so the next morning I received the news that it was a success and that my mother would be back home in a matter of days. When we finally brought her home and I saw her original rosy skin color quickly returning to her face and hands, I knew that the final weights that had been pressed so tightly on me throughout her illness had finally lifted, and that before long, I could begin focusing exclusively on my life once again. Within a month she was back to her usual routines from before her cancer diagnosis and subsequent liver damage had entered her life. Moreover, she was back to her normal behavior, which included pressing me to step up my search for job opportunities and other graduate schools.

With renewed focus and the feeling of liberation shared by my family, I applied to the geography department of my alma mater. I believed that going back to San Francisco State University would be how I could both complete a master's degree and increase my chances of employment in my field. The steps were simple enough: in addition to the usual application requirements of previous academia, grade point average, and letters of recommendation from my undergraduate advisors, I had to pass the Graduate Record Exam (GRE), of which the department informed me that the only section it cared about was the writing portion. While I did not study as intensely as the average graduate school applicant (*i.e., reading the study books cover to cover or take online practice exams*), my faith in my ability to write paid off in the end when my results were sent to me and I scored in the ninety-eighth percentile for the writing section. With that, and my statement of purpose essay, I was certain that not only would I get in, but that being in a familiar place would inspire me to be the active, creative, and successful individual I was all those years ago as an undergraduate.

My faith in my school having my back turned out to be premature and misplaced. The rejection letter was swift and straight to the point: they claimed that there was just too much competition for the available spots in the graduate class for the fall semester. I experienced a wave of depression I had not felt in the last couple of years, not even with everything my mother had been through nor the many rejections I had received from various jobs. For me, this was the straw that broke the camel's back: I had been able to endure the lack of progress I had made in my job searches, the increasingly mundane routines of my theater job, the reality that I would not be able to afford the expense of the previous graduate program that had accepted me, but this was too much. While comforting me, my parents also told me that the notion I had held onto of my alma mater accepting me back into the fold was by no means automatic and that I had been naive to think so. This initially infuriated me, for it sounded as if they had no faith that it would work in my favor from the start. That fury turned back into depression with the realization that I may have put myself into a no-win situation. I had limited my options and expressed doubts and insecurities because of my implicit anxiety of leaving San Francisco again and my inability to think outside the box and be flexible, most likely because of my autism limiting those abilities.

With nothing to turn to, I sank back into my old routines: I swept the floors, served the concessions and sold tickets at the theater, went to the gym with Greg several days a week. But beyond that I wasted the rest of my time with movies, television, and anything else that could distract me from the pain and humiliation of being unwanted in both graduate school and the professional job market. It was only made worse by a major change at the theater: The Sundance Kabuki Cinema, having long served the community with independent films and a customer/employee-centric business model, had been bought out by a corporate chain called Carmike Cinemas. While Sundance continued operating with its name and brand with general oversight from Carmike, the chain itself was swiftly bought out by AMC Theaters, and at that point, we were to be officially incorporated into the chain.

Having already worked for over two years at the Cinemark theater chain in high school, and having borderline anti-corporate views from the years I spent fighting fossil fuel companies and special interest groups, I was not happy with another takeover of an independent chain that served the local population well. Many of my colleagues agreed, and by the time the transition was complete, the vast majority of them, including all of management and the restaurant/bar staff had left, with only me and a handful of coworkers dealing with the changes as best we could. The bright side was receiving my first-ever promotion to crew leader, which was essentially a crew member with certain managerial powers, including being in charge of assigned work stations and directing the daily business of those stations and the people who operated them. For someone with my disability and a history of not being able to climb the employment ladder, it was a major personal achievement. I could finally show that I was capable of handling more responsibilities without the fear of my limitations holding me back. I held this position for about six months.

Around the time of my promotion, I had already decided I needed something more meaningful and engaging to pursue, and I also decided to reapply for graduate school in the spring, hoping that this time, with my established GRE scores and my former department advisors willing to submit letters of recommendation again, I would have a second chance. Also, ever since I had returned from my Birthright trip to Israel, I had been receiving notices about further opportunities in that country, including with a group called Masa that offered connections to various work internships. After some research, I was informed by Masa of several opportunities with different organizations, one of which offered me the opportunity to work in an internship tailor-made for what I wanted to pursue as a career. The Young Judaea program found me several different nonprofits in Israel, of which I chose a nongovernmental organization called EcoPeace Middle East, which functioned as an environmental peacebuilding entity that simultaneously tackled sustainability and water issues while also attempting to advance peace efforts for a two-state solution between Israel and Palestine. At first, I tentatively committed to Young Judaea for its upcoming five-month program in Tel Aviv while secretly hoping that graduate school would come through for me instead. Although the Israel option sounded exciting, I was feeling the familiar anxiety about transitions and newness returning; for the first time in my life I would be flying by myself to a foreign country and living there on my own. I also feared the hostile environment in and around Israel that I knew about and that being developmentally disabled would make it that much harder for me to adjust to a new and disparate place.

For as long as I could, I dragged the process out and patiently waited for the San Francisco State graduate program to get back to me, hoping I would not be rejected a second time. I had prepared for this moment for a long time, saving as much money as I could from the cinema so that I would be able to pay tuition and rent. Interest-free loans from a Jewish organization brought a major boost to my confidence that I could make it work. On paper this seemed like a good plan. At the same time, Masa also told me about scholarships and grants I could apply for as a first-time participant. Masa ended up covering 55 percent of the total program costs after I applied. It was a strange balance for me: providing a plan for how I was going to spend money for graduate school, while realizing I could save myself a substantial amount of money if I committed to Young Judaea. All the while I continued working my cinema job, dealing with numerous crowds of moviegoers, training new recruits every other week, and helping to prepare the theater for the upcoming middle chapter of the Star Wars sequel trilogy. Within a few weeks of the premiere, the decision was finally made.

After waiting several months for an answer, I was informed that once again, my graduate application was rejected, again due to stiff competition. While I was upset and dismayed by the news, I still had a choice to make. Faced with continuing to work indefinitely for a corporate entity I was dissatisfied with, or potentially finding my calling halfway around the world, I paid the program tuition for Young Judaea, along with a plane ticket for Tel Aviv, and subsequently began packing for a journey that would last through the first half of the upcoming year. Despite the continued doubts and anxiety I was feeling about committing to this program for that amount of time, I had to convince myself I had already proved I could tackle major life changes on my own without having my autism hold me back, and that if I could overcome my past struggles, I could certainly make it through this one.

A week after the New Year passed, my father took me to the San Francisco airport. I checked my bags onto the flight and prepared to go through security. Standing there, seeing the path that was laid out ahead of me, I turned to my father, hugging him tightly for about ten seconds that felt more like ten minutes, and told him I would manage as best as I could overseas. He, in turn, thanked me for helping to take care of my mother for the last two years and encouraged me to go find my own life again. He said he would be proud of me no matter what happened. Now feeling assured, I stepped into the security line and, after looking back one last time like I might not see him again, disappeared into the maze of security personnel and machinery.

CHAPTER 22
ANOTHER DOOR OPENS

No one said this journey was going to be easy. That is what I kept trying to convince myself as complications arose from the start of my trip. Getting through security presented no problems; it was at my flight gate where it all began. The moment I arrived I was informed that due to weather conditions and some minor runway issues, my flight was to be delayed by two hours. In the back of my mind, I was hoping this was not a bad omen, for I was already anxious about a number of things already, the biggest of which was how I would be able to handle myself when I eventually made it to Israel all by my lonesome.

After distracting myself as best as I could, I was finally able to board my flight bound for New York where I would transfer to the El Al Israel airline that would take me straight to Tel Aviv. Upon arrival at a heavily snowed-in JFK airport, it became immediately clear that this was the worst possible time to be traveling through the East Coast. The international terminal was crowded, especially around the area where I had to check in for my flight. The news soon got around that there was a slight collision between two aircraft on the runway that, while minimal in damage, had the effect of delaying all outbound flights for upward of five hours. That news, on top of the stringent security measures taken by El Al, was enough to cause my anxiety to spike to near unbearable levels. I never wanted to find myself in a position where I was all alone in an ocean of stranded travelers, having to ferociously guard my luggage and hope that this would not drag on any longer than it had to. Hoping for a smooth transition with few complications and routine boarding procedures turned out to be wishful thinking.

Eventually, after waiting for many hours that stretched my patience far thinner than usual, I managed to get through security and into the terminal where I would board my flight. As it turned out, I was lucky to have gotten through when I did, for shortly after I boarded, a water main broke inside the waiting area where I had spent half the night waiting and flooded the floor I was on moments before. The flight was not an easy one, and I was concerned that when I reached the end of it, I would experience an all-too-familiar feeling. When I had last come to Israel for Birthright, both my circadian rhythm (*the time zone "body clock"*) and my nervous system were affected to the point where I had constant anxiety that made me physically sick and disoriented, and for the first few days my medication had no effect at all. When I arrived at Ben Gurion Airport on the outskirts of Tel Aviv, my fear was confirmed: not only was I beginning to feel the same symptoms as before, but I was informed that my checked luggage never made it onto my flight because of the fiasco at JFK. This news combined with the bad feelings in my system made me agitated, jittery, and sick all at once. But left with no choice, I dragged myself out of the airport and took a cab to a hotel I had booked for several days before I was to move into the apartment that was to be my temporary home. Unable to sleep from the uncomfortable flight and stress over my lost possessions, and with my agitation and shaking getting progressively worse, I called home to let my parents know the situation. While it was difficult to believe them at that moment, they assured me that this event had happened to them and many other travelers too, and since I was assured that my luggage would arrive in the coming days and that I would be whole again by that time, the tiniest bit of relief trickled through me. After that conversation, I managed to force myself to get some much-needed sleep.

Slumber did not last long, however, for at seven in the morning the sound of construction going on next door and of men speaking Hebrew outside my window awakened me. The sound was already loud, but my sensitive hearing made it even more amplified, and the unfamiliar language and voices caused an instantaneous surge of anxiety and fear, the likes of which I had not experienced in many years. My medication (*a combination of anti-anxiety and antidepressants*) once again had no effect on it, and I was tossing and turning in my bed, occasionally clutching my chest because what felt like an air pocket there was constricting my muscles around my heart and near my lungs. If someone had been looking at me from the foot of the bed, they would most likely have thought that I was in the throes of a major drug withdrawal episode. Eventually, my symptoms calmed enough for me to get breakfast. Although I did not feel hungry and knew I had to stay as far away from caffeine as possible, I managed to eat some muffins and have a cup of herbal tea before I decided to go explore the city and make my way toward the beach. Seeing the broad expanse of the sand and the impossible blue of the Mediterranean brought a welcoming sense of relief as my heightened anxiety and chest pains quickly dissipated. I stared out at the water and began walking along the shoreline.

Near the south end of the main beach was a rock formation that stretched several hundred meters into the sea. Fishermen dotted along both sides of the formation and an apparently drunk middle-aged man was jamming out to some Bob Marley tunes on a portable loudspeaker. Despite the slightly treacherous look of the rocks, I needed to find a little adventure to feel more comfortable and alive, so I began carefully climbing the rocks and managed to venture out to the halfway point, which gave me two perfect scenic views, with the sea on one side and the stretch of beach with the many seaside hotels and high-rises dotting the shoreline on the other. In that moment, I felt a sense of peace much like the effect of hours of meditation, which convinced me of the popular belief that the sight and sound of the sea have a calming effect on the body, mind, and soul. When I eventually had to leave the beach, the anxiety I had felt before partially returned, which would compel me to continue visiting the beach over the next few days. The intense symptoms continued to haunt me while I slowly accustomed myself to my new surroundings. This was due in part to the fact that I had only spent one day in Tel Aviv when I was there on Birthright and had only so many familiar places to return to. I did, however, find some comfort when I ran into others who were on their own Birthright trips, and I used the opportunity to encourage them to embrace their Jewish heritage and consider pursuing long-term programs like the one I was about to start. I may not have yet started my Masa program, but I felt obligated to display confidence and excitement despite my anxiety in order to set a good example for them and hopefully excite them to pursue the programs too.

Three days later, it was time to check out of my hotel; I took the few possessions I had with me (*my luggage not yet returned*) and walked twenty city blocks past Bauhaus-style homes, rugged-looking shopkeepers, and busy streets full of buses and Western-made cars to the place I would be calling home for the first half of the year. It was a second-floor apartment above a clothing shop that looked out at a neighborhood full of buildings that had seen better days compared with the ones I was used to back home, with dirty, crumbling walls, air conditioners hanging loosely from balconies, and sidewalks that were barely three feet wide with thick globs of pavement mixed with cobblestones. With that, I placed my stuff in my single bedroom and waited to see what company I would be keeping from then on.

CHAPTER 23
WELCOME TO THE FAMILY

They came in one by one over a span of twenty minutes, and I knew right then that I was going to be in good hands. My three roommates came from all corners of North America: Marcus was a tall, wiry, and slightly unshaven young man with short, sandy-blond hair, and was from Washington DC; Ryan was a bit heavyset and towering with long, hippie-like blond hair, and a natural at-ease demeanor, and he had flown in from Miami; and Ben was shorter and quieter, with brown hair plastered to his head and black-rimmed glasses set into his bookish face, and he hailed from Toronto, Canada. From the onset of the program, they were the coolest, most relaxed, and easiest people to approach that I had ever had the privilege of living with. They laughed at all of my impulsive, situational jokes, were a great help in maintaining the look and feel of a great apartment, and were all-around fun people to spend time with. Our apartment was something all of us treasured: the living room was spacious with a ceiling that rose at least fifteen feet high, we had three bedrooms (*two singles and one double*), two bathrooms, and a kitchen combined with the living and dining room. To me, it was as if I had finally got a place of my own to call home, even if it was only temporary. It felt so good, despite my continued anxiety over being in a foreign country and my still missing luggage, which would be returned later that night. After they were all settled in, we set off into the heart of Florentin, a neighborhood in south-central Tel Aviv, to meet the people who created this program and this major opportunity for us. Once we arrived at the meeting place in a small cultural center, we met the rest of the participants who had flown from all across the world to live and work in the Holy Land.

There were thirty of us in all, and while the majority were Americans like me, there were others from countries such as England, Brazil, and Argentina. To my surprise and comfort, a half-Filipino woman with flowing brown hair named Johanna also came from San Francisco. This made me think that having someone who knows where I come from would help make the transition easier for me, and maybe even for both of us. We then met the people in charge: Tamar Zer-Aviv, the young, hard-headed, yet sharp and enthusiastic program manager for the spring semester of Young Judaea; Dafna Meller, an older, mellow yet well-informed internship coordinator who was the one that arranged my job and everyone else's; and Gili Angert, the brand new program coordinator who would be the one directly in charge of everyone in my program. After several rounds of icebreakers and going over the ground rules of the program, we began our two weeks of orientation, which consisted of activities gauging the importance of our reasons for choosing this program whether it was work experience or making aliyah *(Hebrew for immigrating to Israel)*, a two-day excursion to the Negev desert and the southern city of Eilat, and more than a week of intensive Hebrew courses. I found some of the reasons people gave for coming to this program to be rather amusing, such as one where it was important for one of the women in my group, an Azerbaijani-American woman named Valeriya "Lera" Nakshun, to find a spouse while living here. Most of the other reasons were more serious ones like advancing our career aspirations, which was the primary reason I had chosen to be here.

The trip to the south of the country was a real eye-opener for me. Despite having been there on Birthright, I had never been as far south as we ended up going, nor did I have as immersive of an experience. This time we stayed on a kibbutz, a large collective community rooted in utopian and socialist ideals, and wandered around the massive sand dunes in the desert surroundings in silence in which we could easily meditate. We ended up spending the evening lying out on the kibbutz's soccer field with wine and liquor, watching a clear night sky and stars while waxing poetically about life, liberty, and the pursuit of nonstop fun and experience in a place half a world away from our normal lives in our respective countries.

I very much want to say that everything about this period of time I spent in Israel was as incredible as the night we shared under the stars, but as real life shows, there is always something that makes it more difficult than you would want it to be. That particular difficulty was laid bare in the extreme hardship I had in attempting to learn Hebrew during the intensive language classes, called *Ulpan*, that we had to take during orientation. Having attempted for several years to learn Spanish, with other attempts to master other languages throughout my life, Hebrew brought back a feeling that I knew all too well: the language classes greatly heightened my self-consciousness and made me believe that I was struggling more than the other people in my class. Because of the extreme difficulty of the language; how what I read was written differently than how I would write it, how the Hebrew alphabet was shorter than the English one, writing right to left, and innumerable implied vowels, I came to the same conclusion I had made when I had given up language studies before: that whether my autism had anything to do with it, my brain simply could not process a language different from my own, not to mention that being autistic had already made it difficult for me to understand my native tongue over a number of years.

I eventually decided to discontinue the lessons in favor of focusing on my internship, and everything else about the program I enjoyed more than I can express. I knew it on my first day of work at EcoPeace Middle East. It was a collection of offices that took up the fourth floor of a building used by other businesses and nonprofits, with a view of downtown Tel Aviv that rivaled San Francisco. The staff consisted of a number of people of different nationalities and religions, including expatriate Americans, Israeli citizens, and non-Jewish individuals, which included my direct supervisor, an Italian woman who was in charge of International Affairs for EcoPeace. From the moment I was given my first assignment to create and update a template of every contact EcoPeace had, I knew that I had achieved the one thing I had spent so many years fruitlessly searching for: employment at an organization in my area of expertise. To that end, I worked as hard as I could for them, completing the template within a week. I also attended staff meetings and was given the chance to do research and contribute to an upcoming presentation in London to convince investors to support a project involving several countries in the region.

As I familiarized myself with EcoPeace's work, I began to understand the depth of its mission. EcoPeace had offices in Israel, Jordan, and the Palestinian territories, and the group's mission was to foster cooperation among the countries as a way to prove that peace is possible, using collective participation in grassroots activism, education, and business, specifically through a sustainable business model. In particular, the research I was doing for the presentation was for a project known as the Water-Energy Nexus, which encouraged Jordan to use vast areas of desert land for solar energy development, and using said solar energy to create electricity, some of which would be delivered to Israel and Palestine. In return, Israel would provide Jordan and Palestine with fresh water from its many desalination plants, where it turned saltwater into freshwater to quench the thirst of a vast desert population. Seeing as water is an important resource in many ways, this fit perfectly into what I had been looking for all of this time.

As I got to know the staff, I also made friends with the interns I worked alongside, to the point where they quickly began to spend time with me outside of work and often joined my program friends in various activities. In many ways, I was able to prove to myself that I could combine my professional and personal life without either one overwhelming the other, though in a couple of cases I chose to bring work home with me because of deadlines and my commitment to those tasks. It was not without some complications, for my lack of experience with certain office computer programs and my infrequent bursts of anxiety would sometimes make the tasks more difficult, especially when my supervisor had disagreements about the quality of some of my work. While it often discouraged me in the beginning and even made me question at one point if I was fit to handle the multitasking and quasi-perfectionist nature of the workplace, I eventually came to the conclusion that this was a great learning experience in which having someone as a strong supporter yet occasionally fierce critic would keep me on my toes and make me want to do better for her and the organization.

Through my EcoPeace work, I also began doing two other things simultaneously: proving my worth to them in the hope that they might hire me as a full-time employee and researching the overall Israeli job market to see if the Israeli economy would benefit me better than back home. To that end, I attended several workshops, both in and out of the program, in order to gauge the legitimacy of their operations and hiring capabilities. Israel has been known for a number of things, among them being labeled as a "startup nation" because of the sheer volume of new businesses springing up, and for the encouragement of "Aliyah," or a return to the Holy Land from the diaspora that scattered Jews across the world. If I were to be hired in Israel, I would most likely be achieving both of those aims: living and working for relatively new companies, with the exception of EcoPeace, which had been in existence since I was a toddler. The results were, unfortunately, not what I had hoped for: EcoPeace did not end up hiring me, particularly because it benefited from having a number of interns coming in to work in a revolving door fashion, in addition to a veteran full-time staff with little turnover. Furthermore, I discovered that 12 percent of the working Israeli population was in the tech industry, and that the rest of the country's jobs, colloquially termed as the non-tech industry, had an average salary of slightly less than what I had earned at my previous job at the movie theater, making it difficult for me to live in Tel Aviv.

In what felt like the final nail in the coffin, when I attended a networking event for a startup environmental nonprofit, I was informed that Israeli employers are not only more exacting in their requirements for prospective employees, but that speaking adequate, borderline-fluent Hebrew was an absolute must. While it was disheartening for me to realize I did not have a professional future to look forward to in Israel, it did not stop me from wanting to make the best out of an incredible opportunity I had been given by Young Judaea to live and work in the country. To that end, I resolved to make my overall experience in Israel outweigh any negatives that arose. I wanted to show that, autistic or not, I could be a happy and fulfilled person taking advantage of the fact that I had so many friends, places, and experiences to look forward to in what was shaping up to be the most transformative year of my life thus far.

CHAPTER 24
PARTS IN THE SUM OF THE WHOLE

To say that our bonding experience ended with our orientation and trip to southern Israel would be the worst possible lie I could make up. Over the course of the next five to six months, I got to bond with both my program participants and the Young Judaea staff in ways I would never have thought possible back home. They were quite the mix beyond their different backgrounds. To name a few, Marcus was an architect who had put the practice aside in order to pursue an interest in film production; Ryan was a young progressive who somehow managed to possess an interest in guns, though solely for the use of legal hunting and the shooting range; Antonia was a British national with short brown hair, a posh fashion style, and a sense of adventure who had joined the program because of her sister's prior experience in the program; and Danna, a tall, blonde former-dancer-turned-financial-planner who was to intern with the Israeli branch of Oppenheimer Holdings. While I was by no means friends with everyone, partially owing to the fact that half of them were living an hour away in Haifa, I managed to maintain good relations with the majority of them. In one instance, because one apartment did not like unannounced visits by people staying over from Haifa, my roommates and I opened our doors to them and had a lot more welcome company from that point on.

Never Mr. Life-of-the-Party, I was happy that, unlike in FEMA Corps, I never made any enemies nor did I hold any hard feelings against anyone. While I did not approach certain people because their social temperaments (*passive-aggressive energy, a bit self-absorbed, inability to bond over more than self-interests*) reminded me of people I had a hard time trying to bond with, there were not many of them. Furthermore, by not trying to put myself in potentially awkward situations by not thinking before I spoke or impulsively acting a fool for entertainment, I was able to create an environment where I had plenty of people to comfortably interact with while having enough space from those I could not. I credit part of this with having developed an ability to better read people by the tone of their voice, how they carried themselves, and how open they behaved in their social interactions with others. This was something that does not always come easy for me, and for some on the autism spectrum it does not come at all.

I believe the other part was, quite simply, the fact that the Israeli community was more honest, open, and keen on the concept of straight talk and having intellectually stimulating conversations. I did not come out of my shell quickly, but over time, seeing these interactions and realizing how the Israeli community is so close that it is expected of us to be open to as many people as possible, I began to forge new friendships that felt meaningful to me with many of the local Israelis and foreign expatriates, American and others, with more ease than I had originally thought possible.

One prominent example of making a friend in Israel came from an unexpected source. For a time I shared an office with one of the Israeli employees at EcoPeace, a middle-aged field researcher for the nonprofit, and then one day she told me she had a son my age that she thought I would get along with. This kind of thing had almost never happened to me, not since early childhood. Curious, I accepted her offer to connect us, and within a week I met Shir Tamari at a neighborhood bar around the corner from my house. Like all young men in Israel who are drafted at some point into the armed forces, Shir had the look of a military veteran; he had short black hair halfway between a buzz cut and a summer crew cut, serious brown eyes, slightly grizzled features due to his facial hair, and was tall and fit, with an air of someone who was not to be messed with.

Despite this commanding and intimidating presence, he proved to be welcoming and sociable from the outset, and over the course of four hours, we talked about everything from our personal histories to current events. He worked for cybersecurity most nights of the week, had a father who was an engineer and a sister studying to be one, and lived in a decent, one-bedroom apartment by the Dizengoff Center, one of the most popular shopping centers in Tel Aviv. If this sequence of events had occurred back in the United States, I, like many others, would have found it strange for a woman from work to want to arrange for her grown son to see me and hope we become friends, yet in Israel, it was quite the common occurrence. What did not come as a surprise was how if you met any young Israeli man or woman and got to know them, you would get to know their entire, tight-knit family in short order. When the weeklong Jewish holiday of Passover arrived, my program friends and I were told that it was practically a crime if we didn't spend the first night of celebration, known as the Seder, with an Israeli family, so after asking Shir if I could celebrate with him and his family, he graciously agreed.

While I was initially nervous and concerned that my underdeveloped social skills would show during the Seder dinner, meeting an extended Israeli family was an experience that taught me so many important lessons. After arriving in the nearby town of Ramat HaSharon in the family car, I was introduced to upward of twenty members of the Tamari family, consisting of grandparents, aunts, uncles, cousins, and other distant relatives. The house was situated in a landscape that reminded me of the Spanish countryside I had seen when I spent a summer there with my family years ago, and the house itself was so spacious it could fit an entire unit of soldiers. The table was loaded with plates of braised lamb, bowls of matzah ball soup with shredded egg whites in the broth, loaves of challah, and endless amounts of hummus. During the reading of the story of Moses, while I did not understand Hebrew well, I knew enough to follow along. Afterward, the rest of the night went on with much feasting and conversation. Shir's extended family seemed to like the fact that an American half-Jew like myself was among them, which put me at the center of attention when it came to both practicing their English skills and learning about the differences between their lives and mine back in the United States. No one looked at me like a stranger, and they all treated me with respect and dignity, as I did them. Best of all, no one seemed to be bothered by any of my habits, from impulsive questioning to my facial expressions of confusion and nervousness when Hebrew was being spoken. This made me think that to them, I was just another normal American trying the understand their way of life, albeit with more kindness and an open, inclusive personality compared with the stereotype of loud, awkward, and sometimes ignorant Americans they had heard stories about (*and of which other foreigners I have met in my life have described as well*). After being dropped off by Shir's family at the end of the evening, I concluded that not only did I truly feel comfortable being myself, but I also learned the true value of what being part of a close, extended family was all about. Over the years, my own extended family had become more disconnected to the point where I was only close to my parents.

In the Young Judaea program itself, the excursions and the friends I made from both my program and other Masa programs stood out as the highlights of my entire experience. While my roommates were amazing people, the person who quickly became my best friend was Ellie, a British national studying at a dance studio for her internship. A bespectacled, flamboyant yet fun social butterfly, with an eccentric fashion sense and a crop of short brown hair that at times looked flyaway, she brought out my inner party animal, inviting me to outings with local friends of hers, recommending clubs to check out, and generally being the life and soul of our group. Alternatively, she was a kind and understanding person who was always there for me when I needed her, listened to my long-winded personal stories, and challenged me to look beyond my social ineptitudes and relax into myself and the new environment I was in. I had to constantly remind myself how incredibly lucky I was to have a friend like her, and I believe that she felt the same way, as she trusted me with her personal stories and insecurities. She went out of her way to be a constant, supportive presence in my life, and I was there to help her whenever she was dealing with her personal dramas. While this may seem like a typical discovery of someone who became my best friend, being autistic, it was anything but, for this was the first time in nearly four years I had someone to call a best friend. It was also the first time in several years that someone genuinely wanted to be in my social life all the time. Most importantly for me, it was the first time since middle school where someone checked in with me on her own accord more times than I did on her, for in the majority of my friendships, I had long felt that I was always the one who put in more effort and interest.

Despite living in the far north of Israel, I also managed to make good friends with several of the Haifa program members, which included Vasily, a tall, fit, and blond German national of Russian descent who documented our adventures throughout the semester while wearing his signature summer vacation attire; Benjamin, a shorter yet robust New Jersey native of Puerto Rican descent with a big personality that was also as flamboyant as Ellie's; and Will, a towering yet fun-loving and grizzly-faced Brazilian national who laughed at all of my ridiculous situational jokes.

About halfway through the program, I was given the opportunity to apply for a leadership academy training session in Jerusalem, which I was accepted into and spent a week at a hotel on a kibbutz overlooking a large section of the holy city. While I was there, I learned a number of things about how to be an effective leader in an abstract fashion; in other words, I had to determine how to be a leader with no specific situation to apply those skills to. While it was frustrating at first, it did teach me important lessons, such as the difference between adaptive leadership, which involves people and requires learning, and technical leadership, in which an expert is involved and the solution is already known. From there it was about how to find the best possible way forward with the people I was assigned to work with, observing their behaviors and interactions, interpreting the various positions and viewpoints, and intervening if disagreements and frustrations boiled over.

As a person with autism, these concepts proved difficult for me to comprehend. One prominent reason was the lack of an example of a specific situation for either type of leadership. I had long been able to understand how to solve problems and take a leadership role if I knew what kind of situation I was dealing with. With no examples or concepts to go on, I was drawing a blank on how to apply it and work with my group. Tied in with my lack of comprehension was a feeling of implicit anxiety; while I did not show symptoms like panic attacks or fidgeting, the anxiety nonetheless affected me in a way that was only remedied by staying silent while my group debated steps to address abstract leadership skills. One advantage I had, however, was feeling the need to maintain order and harmony in the group; when frustrations were aired, I felt the impulse to step in and calm the situation to allow for further debate and problem-solving. Soothing tensions gave me relief as well, for arguing and constant loud noises fed my anxiety, even when I was taking my antidepressant medication. Through this experience, I learned that while I was not able to directly contribute to being an abstract leader, I served an important function as a team player through helping my group keep cool heads, which allowed us to move along and work together to the end of the exercise. In a way, serving in this function made me feel like I was a leader through my contribution, and that we were all leaders in our own right in how we all moved as cogs in a machine.

During that time, I made friends with many more people from the various programs Masa had, which included Israel Teaching Fellows, Career Israel, and even a teaching credential program designed specifically for Russian nationals. Among the friends I made were Miranda, a fellow San Francisco Bay Area native, with the kind of quasi-bohemian fashion sense I was used to back home; Roy, another American, with dark, curly hair and glasses who happened to live in the same Tel Aviv neighborhood as me; and Roni, a wiry-looking Israeli with matted black hair and pointed facial features who came from the south near Gaza and who proved to be a lively individual. Together, we worked through our workshops and became close through networking and sharing similar interests, culminating in the Masa Gala in downtown Jerusalem where everyone saw me break out into the hip-hop dancing I loved. Throughout the night, the reaction I got from everyone through dance was positive, even more so when, to my great surprise, I got to dance with one of the Russian women in the group who looked like a model from a Victoria's Secret runway. Having danced solo my entire life, the pure ecstasy of having a beautiful woman in my arms, stepping in rhythm seamlessly without crushing each other's feet as half of the gala watched us, was one of the most wonderful feelings in the world. I was feeling like the luckiest, most normal, fun-loving person in the room. By the end of the training, I not only had learned new leadership skills, but had managed to be my true self and make new friends who wanted to spend more time together when the next opportunity arose.

The excursions Young Judaea provided for us proved to be far more in-depth and educational than what I had previously experienced in the Birthright program. On nearly every Tuesday throughout my time in Israel, I either visited various cities, towns, and sites around the country or took part in charitable acts of assistance around Tel Aviv alongside my friends and fellow participants. From the long hike along the Ein Gedi Plain and Oasis to the visit we paid to the ethnic Druze village of Beit Jann in the mountains of northern Israel, every experience made me feel like not only was I embracing the multicultural aspects of the country, but that we, as a program group, were embracing it together, making us that much closer friends.

At the helm of nearly every trip we took was Gili, who made sure that she was the most present figure in our lives and wanted us to know that not only was she the one who put this together for us, but that it was as much an adventure for her as it was for us. For example, we went to a low-key shopping center combined with a major bus station in Tel Aviv where we were asked to help with cleaning out a junk-filled room in preparation for converting it into a daycare center for toddlers, mostly immigrant and other minority children whose parents could not afford other centers. Clearing out junk, rearranging useful furniture, and scaring the roaches out of corners proved to be a time of great camaraderie for

Gili, my colleagues, and me. Some of them worked with kids for their internships and Gili had a background in social work, and for me, it brought back memories from when I interned at UC Berkeley and educated children in spaces a lot like the one we were in. When we saw another daycare center in the same mall being used by the type of kids we were preparing the other room for, we all felt a sense of validation for the work we put into preparing that space, and the comfort in knowing that we would bring much-needed support to the families of Tel Aviv.

Gili and I had a special relationship from the start of the program. In the first week she insisted on getting to know us one-on-one and invited us to a neighborhood coffee shop so she could see how best to support us. When it came my turn I was almost as nervous as when I had lost my luggage at the airport. To me, this was all too familiar from when I had my one-on-one with J.T., and how she went from a seemingly compassionate woman to an abusive monster, and I was fearful of the same thing happening here. With her long, light-brown hair gently flowing down her shoulders, her friendly brown eyes staring deep into mine, and a small, genuine smile playing around her lips, Gili started off with technical questions, asking me why I chose to be in the program and what I hoped to accomplish. I gave her answers that ranged from work experience to seeing if this would be a place for me to live one day. When she came to the question of what kind of person I saw myself as, I hesitated. I could hear my father's voice in my head telling me "It's OK to tell the truth, but you shouldn't always tell the whole truth." What could I tell her? Should I cover up my social ineptitudes and present myself as a confident, well-put-together young man? Should I change the subject? Should I gloss over weaknesses and focus only on strengths? I could not decide. So I told her I was not sure how to describe myself because I am afraid to let people know about me, owing to the fact that I consider myself a bit different and that many people do not like different. It was then that she told me of her degree in social work and how she had always felt it was important for everyone to be their true self no matter what, something, she added, that has always been celebrated in Israel. She further revealed that compared with the average Israeli woman, she always considered herself as kind, considerate, sensitive, and open, whereas most other women were more strong-willed, hard-headed, and protective of themselves until others got to know them. It was because of her moment of vulnerability that I decided to take the chance and tell her about my *true* self. Upon hearing the details of my autism, she declared that just by being brave and open, I proved I had a kind heart and that she would always be there for me if I needed anything. From then on we were close, whether it was updating her on the progress in my internship or stepping up to defend her when some people in the program gave her a hard time over roommate issues or a perceived lack of accommodations and assistance.

Perhaps the most impactful experience of my time in Young Judaea took place outside of Israel, when I was accepted into a Masa delegation of about forty participants to travel to Poland for a week in order to visit Holocaust sites and meet with Jewish leadership in Krakow and Warsaw. It was particularly important to me because most of my father's Jewish family members have their roots in Poland, but since they left long before the events of the second World War, I was to be the first member of my family to set foot there in more than 150 years. To make it even more meaningful for me was a question I carried with me as we flew north toward Europe: after all of the most unimaginable horrors of the Holocaust, how was it not a cultural black hole for the Jewish community? That question was answered swiftly when we arrived in Krakow, a city of ancient and classic Polish architecture stretching back to medieval times that was largely spared from the violence of the war, albeit still impacted by the deportation of Jews to concentration camps. Upon meeting representatives at the Jewish Community Center, we learned that many Jews, Polish and foreign alike, were participating in what they called a "Jewish Revival" in which they would welcome anyone with any amount of Jewish ancestry into the fold in an effort to recreate the once vibrant culture that flourished in the days of pre-war Poland. Our subsequent meeting with a Holocaust survivor shed even more light upon the revival efforts. She had been robbed of certain experiences as a Jew during the Holocaust, had actively served the remnants of the Jewish community in the postwar era, and was finally able to go through rites of passage, such as a long-delayed Bat Mitzvah ceremony at the tender age of eighty-one. Perhaps the most shocking revelation was the complete lack of anti-Semitic violence in more than three decades, which to me, showed that there was hope for the recovering Jewish population.

Warsaw was a completely different story: the city had been mostly leveled by the Nazis during the war, and was rebuilt during the Cold War when the Soviet Union incorporated the country into its communist empire. As a result, there were only a few reminders of what the ghettos had been like there, with certain buildings either converted into private residences or slated for eventual demolition. Nevertheless, there were a number of memorials and a few preserved building sites to memorialize the plight of the ghetto residents, as well as a Jewish history museum dating back to before medieval times when Jews were seen as vital to the then-kingdom of Poland and under personal protection from the king himself. In between the sites, I bonded with my fellow representatives, many of whom I had met previously at the Jerusalem Leadership Academy, doing everything together from exploring the city and parklands to eating out at Polish restaurants with plenty of pierogies (*a Polish staple*) to go around. Once again, I found that I was able to be myself around them, making great situational jokes, while also being able to have deep conversations about life and current events, and even showing my dancing abilities to general amusement and surprise by those that had not seen me dance before. It was what happened outside of both cities, however, that ironically would have the most profound impact of all.

Inevitably, we made our way to the concentration camps, the first being Auschwitz-Birkenau, an hour outside of Krakow. It was not easy for any of us, most of all me, as we slowly approached the barbed wire fence which ran along the right side of the entrance with the infamous Arbeit Macht Frei (*Work Sets One Free*) sign looming over us. Going through the camp, seeing the personal effects preserved in many of the buildings, having to look at the piles of discarded shoes, luggage, and, dare I say, hair that was cut off all prisoners, was extraordinarily difficult to stomach, to the point where I was a bit concerned about being sick in the middle of the museum. It only got worse from there, seeing the faces of the victims on the walls, watching videos of survivors recounting the horrors of the camp, and eventually, walking into a dark room that had multiple projectors showing the lives of whole families before they were murdered in Auschwitz, along with massive volumes of books that contained the names of those identified from the camp. While I did not openly cry or end up being sick like some of my friends, I was deeply shaken by what I had seen and remained silent for a couple of hours after we had left the camp. For much of my life, I had heard the stereotypes of how people with autism do not have the ability to show, much less feel, strong emotions in situations where they should. While the more ignorant types of people buying into that stereotype might have drawn that conclusion about me if they had been there, they would have been dramatically wrong. I fully believe that while grief can be contained, it can still be felt and shown in different ways, hence the common adage that everyone grieves in their own way. In my case, I sat in silence until we left the camp and found a wide, grassy field to eat lunch, at which point we all began making attempts at conversation about anything other than what we had just been through.

For all of the horrors we witnessed enshrined in Auschwitz-Birkenau, it did not end there. When we traveled outside of Warsaw on our way to the Treblinka extermination camp, we first stopped by the nearby Łopuchowo Forest, which was the site of a major massacre and mass grave created by the Nazis' summarily executing Jews from nearby Tykocin. While I managed to maintain my composure despite the sickening story I heard about a survivor of the massacre, it became too much for one of the women in our group, who walked away to sit by a nearby tree and needed to be consoled by several other members of our group. Seeing her in such a state of emotional pain, the tears running down her face and her face bloated and red from crying so hard quickly became too much for me to bear. So for the rest of the trip, I stayed by her side, doing everything I could to cheer her up, assisting her with whatever she needed, and just simply being a presence that she could find comfort and trust in. A common belief is that autistics do not feel empathy for others. But I did, and do. In Poland, having someone like that to support certainly helped both of us as we fought to keep our composure at Treblinka and during our debrief after we arrived back in Warsaw. Shortly afterward our week came to an end, and we had to make our way back to Israel, but through our shared experiences we had bonded so much more than we did before we arrived in Poland. Through that camaraderie we came back as stronger, wiser, and better people.

If anything, both while in Jerusalem and Poland, I bonded with more people than I ever could have imagined compared with being back home, and their solidarity with me showed when we had several parties and barbecues during Israel's seventieth independence day celebrations and at Masa reunions over subsequent weeks. Having to go through so many difficult situations, only to come out clean on the other side with so many good people added to my corner, brought me to the conclusion that whatever my personal struggles, the sum total of my experiences was worth every moment, no matter how I felt at those times, and that my autism no longer defined who I was, for if anything, it was just a component in making me who I am.

CHAPTER 25
CLOSING THE BOOK TO ADVENTURE

We all knew it was coming, but for some of us, it did not make it hurt any less. The end of the program was upon us, and having already finished our internships and taken our final excursion to the aforementioned Druze village, staying at a hostel near the Sea of Galilee, and rafting down the Jordan River that was made more special for me by sharing my raft and adventure with a free-spirited Gili, we headed to the Young Judaea offices for our graduation ceremony. As we rode the bus to the offices, which were surprisingly close to where I worked, I looked back on closing the chapters of the multifaceted book I had written for myself, starting with the small but significant office party my colleagues had put together as a proper farewell. While I was casual about saying goodbye, deep down I wished that I could have stayed longer, for this was the kind of work I had so fruitlessly tried to find back home. I felt I had proven myself to them, so much so that I wanted very much to work for them full-time. At the least, I now had the real-world experience I believed I so desperately needed, along with references and a letter of recommendation from both my supervisor and the head of the Israel office, which I believed would work wonders as I searched among possible work opportunities with connections to EcoPeace. I visited as many locations in Tel Aviv as I could, from my favorite eateries to the beaches I had swum in, but I still felt like I should have spent more time at these places. I had also made the best of my time with the local Israeli friends I had made, along with the friends I made in Masa. Now it had all come down to this: traipsing up the stairs to the third floor of a white-washed, slightly run-down building into a spacious room where the ceremony was to begin.

Gili, Tamar, and Dafna began the ceremony, which at first consisted of interdepartmental congratulations and a slideshow of our adventures as the Young Judaea Spring Class of 2018. It was also announced, to our collective dismay, that Gili was to depart Young Judaea, citing work stress and an interest in pursuing other things in life. I was particularly saddened by this, having seen how she went out of her way to give us the best experience we could have and how she wanted us to see her not as a boss but as a friend we could always count on. I still hoped she would continue to do great things with her life. It was at that point that we were to make speeches of our own. Gili had approached Marcus and me beforehand to ask if we would speak on behalf of all participants. I agreed enthusiastically. The group knew me as someone who knows a lot of things in general, but what they did not know was that I had an affinity for memorizing historical quotes, and I used one now: the astronomer and philosopher Galileo once said "All truths are easy to understand once they have been discovered, the point is to discover them." I told them I liked to believe that they had done the same for themselves, whether it was in their work, their social interactions, or even in love, and whether they considered their discoveries to be *a* truth or *the* truth from their perspectives. I finished by saying that my truth was how I had never imagined before this that I would feel so fulfilled in my professional and personal life, nor that I would have a group of friends and a helpful staff that became an extended family in the process, and that while I looked forward to going home, it would be just as hard for me to leave Israel and the life I had cultivated for myself with all of them.

After the speeches, we went to the rooftop for a barbecue. It was also where I would have to say goodbye to my friends from Haifa, so I made the best of my time with them, reminiscing over our adventures, making my Brazilian friend Will laugh some more, and making sure I was someone they would never forget, seeing as I would never forget them. Saying goodbye, while bittersweet, made me happy knowing they thought highly of me, with several of them saying they planned to visit me when they could. Lera, the woman who wanted to make Aaliyah and find an Israeli husband in the process, told me I was a uniquely special and kind person and that I should never stop being myself for anything or anyone.

Finally, I spoke to Gili. Knowing her intention to leave Young Judaea, and being concerned she would think she had not accomplished much in her time with us, I told her about my time in the FEMA Corps. I described how brutal it was for me, and because of the cruelty I experienced at the hands of J.T., I was not convinced at first that I should even be in the Young Judaea program for fear that history would repeat itself. She changed all of that for me, I told her, and she was everything that J.T. never was, and so much more. While I can never truly be sure if my words convinced her, from her reaction alone, I know that at least with me, it validated everything she had done for us and would hopefully make her feel like she accomplished something in spite of the stress and challenges she had faced in her role.

On my last day I was with Antonia at the Jaffa Lookout Point, enjoying one last look at the skyline of the city that had become my spiritual home, a place where I hoped to return one day. The buildings were not the skyscrapers of New York, nor were they quite like the expanses of interconnected cities and towns that made up the San Francisco Bay Area, but this foreign landscape no longer felt like uncharted territory. I could make out the DNA spire-shaped Azrieli Sarona Tower, the Coliseum-like Azrieli Center with its interconnected towers sprouting up on three sides of the central shopping mall, the great highway that bisected the central urban neighborhoods in the west from the sprawling residential areas to the east, and best of all, the curve of the beaches that comprise the eastern end of the Mediterranean Sea, stretching beyond the northern horizon and extending south to the base of the lookout. I could hear the sounds of the city, the laughter and conversations taking place down the hill, the honking of cars and buses, and the waves crashing against the rock wall where the beach ended at the hill. Seeing, hearing, and feeling all of the sights, sounds, and vibrations of this wondrous city, and with Antonia sitting with me, looking so beautiful in her pink and white sundress with her long, flowing brown hair, gave me the kind of peace I had only felt once before when I had attempted to calm myself at the start of the trip. This time, it was not just the water in the sea, it was the symbiotic relationship of the land, the water, the culture, and the beautiful people I had gotten to know who gave me a sense of belonging, that finally helped me find true happiness away from all I knew back home, and where I had made a new home, one that I would without a doubt miss terribly.

Antonia and I had gotten close during the program, and while I was going home, she was not done traveling yet and had many more adventures planned. We talked about the places she would go, from a cross-country trip through Europe to the Arabian Desert. We talked about the work she would do, which involved seeking employment with a communications company and using that to see even more of the world. Lastly, we talked about staying in touch and remaining as close friends. I had confided in her about my autism near the beginning of the program, and instead of rejecting me and pulling away, she surprised me by believing I was a kind, gifted, and intelligent man who deserved to be surrounded by people who cared about me, and through that statement, our friendship grew exponentially. As the late afternoon sun began to sink toward the west, we headed back to our respective apartments for final inspection, where I gave Gili a final gift of chocolate almond bark, courtesy of my mother's special recipe, as she reviewed the state of our living space.

Early the next morning, the time had finally come. With my bags packed and my taxi soon to arrive, I shared one last goodbye with my roommates, who were staying in Israel a bit longer, with the promise that we would see each other again soon and then headed out to the sidewalk where my taxi arrived. As we drove through the city, I took one last look at all of my surroundings: the curvy mismatched streets; the run-down shops with the owners setting up for another day at work; the hummus shops also readying for business by setting up tables indoors and out; the mostly young Israeli citizens walking around the city, many of them in military uniforms to indicate their draft service; and the skyscrapers that made up the Azrieli Sarona Tower, the Azrieli Center, and the Shalom Tower, to name a few. Finally, the driver arrived at the international terminal of Ben Gurion Airport, which I remembered from having gone through it while leaving the Birthright program two years ago.

The departure area was nowhere near as crowded as I thought it would be, perhaps because it was the start of summer and most people would probably want to stay and enjoy the Israeli sun and beaches than travel elsewhere. After checking my bags and being cleared by security, I found myself in a circular waiting area and shopping center. About ninety minutes before I had to board my flight, I went to the food court, bought lunch, and picked a seat with a view of a distant suburb of the Tel Aviv metro area. While staring into the distance, I reflected on all I had accomplished and how I believed it could assist me going forward in life. I would be lying if I were to say that I now had everything figured out, for like before there was a lot of uncertainty on the horizon. Would my work in Israel be enough to convince employers to finally give me a chance? Would I have the strength to push forward if I continued to face stiff resistance on the work front? Would that strength also translate into making a home for myself when I returned? And most of all, would my experiences of acceptance and inclusion in Israeli society finally be mirrored back in the United States so I could feel like I was just another one of the guys?

I came to the conclusion that it probably would not, as life was never that black and white for me then nor now. Therefore, I had to be ready to fight for the life I wanted to live with renewed determination and resolve. My experiences in Israel were proof I do have the ability to make a life for myself and my being disabled didn't have to get in the way of making that a reality. This adventure brought many new people, colleagues, and friends into my life along with their faith and support in me, and this is what I had to carry with me back home, along with all of the other experiences I had that made a positive impact. Having also witnessed the tight-knit nature of an

Israeli family, I also resolved to be a much closer and more helpful son to my parents and to be more in touch with my extended family, wanting to have good relations with them as I saw with Shir's family. To me, my life would always be in flux if I did not make for a good home life to complement whatever career I eventually managed to pin down. Everything else would fall into place as long as I kept busy and accepted my autistic life for what it was, while also striving for what it could be.

I ambled to the departure gate, where I saw a short, brunette woman whom I recognized as Rachel, another one of my program participants, who had coincidentally chosen the same departure flight. As it turned out, we would touch down together in New York before she would make her way to another flight that would take her home to her native Louisiana. Any and all apprehension I had for the flight back was now gone, as I could relax knowing that not only was I going home, but I would have a familiar face with me for the journey across the Mediterranean and the Atlantic. The boarding calls began, and I happened to be one of the last groups to board, which did not bother me because I had so little to carry on. As the line dwindled, I asked myself one final question: would I truly be alright when I arrived in the San Francisco apartment I shared with my family? I decided that there was no easy answer to that, but this different, yet normal, individual would figure it out all in due course. Satisfied with my own answer, I took one last look at the horizon that was Tel Aviv and the State of Israel, and with lingering reluctance, boarded my flight home.

CHAPTER 26
THERE IS NO END, ONLY NEW BEGINNINGS

I cannot be entirely sure where I first heard this saying, only that I was a kid at the time and it has stayed with me ever since. At my lowest points and my greatest highs, that aphorism was always there for me, and even if I did not remember it there and then, I would feel compelled to move on and in some cases, start over, even if it took me a long time to get there. If not for that saying and the accompanying compulsion to move forward, I would not have had as many experiences as I have up to this point, nor would I most likely have had the desire to keep living my life.

Every time I begin again, the thought also crosses my mind that somewhere around the world, whether in my country or another, someone, perhaps more than one, may have just decided that their end has arrived. Perhaps someone has decided it for themselves, or life is so consistently difficult that they feel there is no hope for them to be themselves and to live a life similar to their mainstream, "normal-brained" counterparts. Turning on the news or reading it from my computer, despite the news media's affinity for concentrating on the negative instead of the positive, I cannot help but pay close attention to stories of people who are simply different from others in looks, behavior, or both who end up becoming victims of violent attacks and/or are shunned by whole communities, sometimes even their families. I've also seen negligence and abuse by parents or guardians who snapped under the pressure of caring for a special needs child. Some of these stories never make national news, but I have seen them on local news and sometimes gossip websites, often wishing that they would be given the wider coverage they need.

To me, these stories, among other events, paint an all-too-clear picture of the major stigma attached to mental illness and developmental differences, with many in the present sociopolitical climate enforcing that stigma through quick judgment and oversimplifying how society should work according to their collective beliefs. Hate groups, ranging from neo-fascists to other forms of alt-right groups, further cement these sentiments and instill a general fear of intolerance and brutality. For someone like me, a person on the spectrum, it is scary to think that history could repeat itself, especially after what I witnessed during my trip to Poland. The lesson we learned was put in simple terms: Never Again. Even if I were not Jewish, I have no doubt I would have fallen under the category of *invalide*, used by the Nazis for those either crippled or disabled and therefore not in line with their idea of a "perfect" society. Seeing the rhetoric used in everything from the right-wing rallies to being mocked and implied at the presidential level, my old ultrasensitive and anxious self would impulsively come to the conclusion that it is the end of the world as we know it.

However, there are two distinct differences now: I am older and wiser than I once was, and even though I am well aware that life is not like a movie where the hero ultimately defeats the villain every time, I fully believe in the power and triumph of the human spirit. If people were able to see, regardless of whatever perceived shortcomings they have, the true power they possess, they could well shift the balance of power away from the few that feed off of weakness, misery, and divisiveness to cement a social order of their choosing.

This potential reality, however, cannot occur until others begin to see how important it is to treat autistics, people with mental disabilities, and social introverts as equals, to remind us that we are more than the sum of our development, and to find our niche in our communities where we can prove that we can achieve our dreams and contribute to a more forward-thinking society. For many, it starts with family. I truly would not be who I am today without my family, with parents who, despite occasional frustrations with me, never lost their patience and never stopped encouraging me to be my best self. They provided me with a good life full of experiences, bonding, and the development of a capable, hard-working individual. If parents could look at their child with this positivity, regardless of ability or disability, I truly believe that every individual on earth will find their purpose and live their best lives as a result of the love and support that was bestowed upon them early on.

The process then moves on to friends, employers, and the average person you meet on the street. I believe the biggest obstacle we face as autistic people is not our own limitations but the neurotypical world. Contemporary American society is so fast-paced, so centered on one's own ambition and achievements that it's much easier to label someone you encounter with a disability as "weird" and move on, rather than react to them with curiosity and compassion. From middle school to the adult world, I've experienced this attitude and its resulting behavior — from rejection in the job market and even personal rejection among some members of my extended family — to outright hostility. This is one of the toughest lessons of all, because even for the most optimistic individuals, the reality is that there will always be someone who will never truly accept you for who you are, to the point where antagonism, and sometimes even violence, may occur. It is the worst part of growing up, but in some ways it is also the best: by getting to know who someone truly is, you can learn to let go of the negative influence of those who mean you harm and see who your true friends are. It can be a bitter pill to swallow, as I have experienced on countless occasions, especially when some kind of relationship has been established before it falls apart; however, time has shown me that the right people come along in life when you need them, and a solid community arises for you. The positive ripple effect also happens in the job market, when employers realize they need bright young minds and fresh eyes to advance their objectives, and the more different you are, the better. Most of all, when simple acts of kindness are given to others, whether you know them or not, those acts are either reciprocated or paid forward.

Without any doubt the toughest lesson of all is when the process moves to self-examination. Even for people like me who love ourselves enough to keep living, life can be blind, unintentionally or otherwise, to whatever faults we may possess. As far as I know, there is no one alive or has lived on this planet that has been a "perfect" human being in every way, shape, or form. Our faults are what make us human, though it can often be a tricky process to determine if they are something we can live with or something we either need to work on or get help for. The latter action was a particularly tough one for me because of my constant state of denial through adolescence. I believed that whatever faults I had, I could live with them and not give up any sense of self or independence. Time, encouragement, and the occasional revelation eventually brought me to the point where I not only embraced my faults, but I found the help I needed to make my life better and more enjoyable.

It was also during this time I made another discovery: no two individuals with autism are the same. While it is true we fall under the same classification, somewhere on the spectrum, some of us communicate better than others, some are more obsessed with keeping routines than others, and some are more brilliant in certain areas of knowledge and study than others. We are not all savants like the main character in *Rain Man*. While there may not be any one way to help someone with a social disorder, the fact of the matter is that we are very real, functional, and impressionable human beings, even if our behaviors do not always match the societal definition of "normal."

I have come to the conclusion that there is never truly an end, not even when our time on Earth eventually comes to pass. As long as we are alive, the triumphs, adversities, and other moments represent chapters of our lives where one ends and another begins. Most of these chapters start or end depending on our choices, but our behaviors, abilities, and situations also influence certain outcomes and events we experience throughout the course of our life story. Even after our time has come to an end, many of us leave behind those who will remember us for how we wrote the story of our lives, and hopefully, they attempt to honor that story as best as they can. It is these moments that should inspire us—autistic or not—to live more positive lives and make ourselves and everyone around us happy, while keeping in mind that the reality of our lives involves overcoming adversity and dealing with people who may never understand us and do not deserve us. In my experience, when you think you can solve your own problems and try to make peace with the people and events in your lives that made things difficult for you, it can often be hard to accept that not only will some things never change but that there are always going to be forces beyond your control. It is a bit humbling, for it shows how we are part of something bigger than ourselves and that we need to find a way to be ourselves while also contributing to the world and how it should be with enough belief, tolerance, and hard work.

Whether being autistic or not, smart or clueless, sensible or senseless, I would never assume to be someone who has all of the answers. No one does, whether they are like me, or higher and lower on the spectrum, or those who do not have a single affliction of the mind, body, or soul. I only know what I have learned from my experiences and from those I've known along the way, and how I interpret the world around me. I know the life lessons instilled in me from my parents, teachers, and those I looked up to as role models, and I remember all of the times when I finally opened myself up to knowing more about me and what I was truly capable of.

While I may not function in the same way as many in this country and beyond, I do share many attributes of my neurotypical counterparts: I feel strong emotions, I yearn for adventure, I enjoy television as equally as I like to play ultimate frisbee, I believe strongly in being close to my family and being loyal to my friends, and most of all, I one day want to have a life with a family of my own so I can be even a fraction of as good a parent as mine were to me. I will not let my disability define me for the rest of my life, nor do I want others to believe that either, for me or for themselves. We all have a chance at a happy, fulfilling life, and maybe some of us will achieve it with ease, maybe others, like myself, need to fight a bit harder to get there, but never for a moment do I believe that it is an impossible dream.

Every time it felt like my life was over, another door opened up and compelled me to travel through it; I have met others with my condition who have claimed to have experienced the same. To me, this signifies the start of a new chapter, whether voluntary or forced upon myself. As I fly back to the United States, fresh from closing the chapter of my Israel adventure, I try to think of everything that got me there and what it could mean for my future. My ultimate conclusion is that while I have no overall control over what comes next, and my personal history dictates that adversity will remain, I will always manage to overcome it in the end, and with every trial and tribulation conquered, life will become easier and more meaningful. So, too, begins another of the many new beginnings for me, and I hope, for anyone else who lives in a society where living beyond the definition of normal exists, and that could never—and will never—limit us as human beings.

ACKNOWLEDGEMENTS

American poet Haniel Long once wrote "So much of what is best in us is bound up in our love of family, that it remains the measure of our stability because it measures our sense of loyalty." Throughout my story I have detailed what I believe to be a straightforward, unflattering account of my life as an autistic individual, whether or not I acknowledged it at the time. Through that story I have highlighted every person who had a significant impact on my life, for good or ill. While those who treated me as less than their equal and those whose privacy is my primary concern, will remain anonymous beyond their initials, it would be fundamentally wrong of me to not highlight those who helped me embrace my abnormalities and turned them into something to celebrate. The acts of kindness, understanding, and loyalty I have received have shaped my perspective in such a way that while I do have many people whom I consider to be my friends, I also believe that the term "family" is more relative than it sounds; there are those who showed so much care and understanding when I needed it the most that I wish they were a part of my family. I give special thanks and recognition to the following:

— Erin Gruwell: Freedom Writer teacher, nonprofit founder, and personal friend, who inspired me to always see with my heart and to write what needs to be written.

— Molly McClure: One of the first people to be unconditionally kind to me as a child, proving that memories and good vibes can still be felt many years later.

— Mrs. Chantal Mace (nee Ms. Lacrampe): For seeing and believing in the potential I possessed, one of the first to recognize what a "big heart" I had, and for being my biggest supporter as a child in her classroom; a catalyst for my future good deeds and how I saw myself in later life.

— Brett Olson: For having a constantly fun and positive outlook on life and surprising me by doing things for me and seeing me the way many people in school never did; unfortunately passed away eight years before the writing of this memoir, may God rest his soul.

— Christina "Tina" Pinedo: For showing me kindness, tolerance, and solidarity; bonding with me through mutual trust and shared interests; and for being a tireless supporter and campaigner for disability rights everywhere.

— Joshua Moldoff: For being a consummate friend and supporter, loving every story I told, and being one of the first to say that he looked up to me.

— Elizabeth "Liz" Blee: For allowing me to be your first "patient" in your path to becoming a psychologist; showing unbelievable patience, understanding, and maturity beyond your years; and for being my rock in the stormy seas of high school and beyond.

— Jordan Fillmore and Joey Anderson: The basketball team captains who genuinely appreciated my school spirit and admiration for them as players and people; treated me with the same kindness and respect I gave to them.

— Jenny Reich: For her endless, selfless encouragement, and for molding me into an effective speaker and debater in Model United Nations; a catalyst for my development in public speaking.

— Kanika Patel: For making our walks home from school fun; for being so wise, mature, and easy to talk to; and for giving me the Senior Ball experience I thought I would never have.

— Mr. Bob Barter: For challenging me to think outside the box, for being a great teacher, and for being the kind of person you felt so blessed to call your mentor when good people like him were in such short supply.

— Rikki Shackleford: For blessing me with the opportunity to work for the University of California, Berkeley, Lawrence Hall of Science and expanding my knowledge and perspectives on environmentalism, community service, and cultivating the minds of children in our society.

— The TEAMS program: For blessing me with opportunities to give back to the community through education and community, and for providing me with a team of amazing friends; special shout-out to Mariah, Isaac, and Cimone Fowler, Chris and Andrew Clausen

— Lana Husser: For creating and running a truly revolutionary environmental media program, The Green Screen, giving me the chance to be an effective reporter and a good citizen to the people of Richmond, and for allowing me to be my parents' son in their field of work.

— Tyler Jolley, James Wiley, and Josh Martarella: My main crew in the Green Screen, who shared all of my interests, fully accepted me and my odd habits, and made for a special kind of camaraderie as we documented and assisted in changing the lives of our community for the better; special shout-out to the rest of the Green Screen, who made the dream even more real and worth living—Doug Scott, Joaquin Navas, Andrew Balderas, Kelly Saefong, Celiana Sanchez, and Morgan Valdevieso, to name a few!

— Brian, R.J., and Alodie Crizaldo: For dedicating your lives to a community that needed you, for helping to pass on the experiences of the hip-hop community to others that needed it, and for including me in your incredible family of dancers, artists, and all-around selfless people!

— John Michael "J.M." Salvatierra: The nephew of hip-hop royalty, who immediately accepted me as a friend and whom I could not be more blessed to have in my life, and whom I credit with having the best experiences outside of my "bubble" of a town; special recognition to fellow friends Cameron Lee and Mikela Padilla.

— R.J. "Kool Raul" Navalta: The man who helped bring glory to the Bay Area by bringing our hip-hop dance culture to the national stage and who selflessly mentored and supported me in the beginning of my foray into the hip-hop community; I'm proud to this day to call you my brother, for you truly are the surrogate big brother I wish was part of my family; for saving my life in more ways than one.

— Taeko McCarroll: Another hip-hop great, the first to give me a chance to work in a passion field of mine when no one else would, went beyond a boss and friend to become a surrogate big sister whom I am beyond blessed to have in my life and who, in many ways, strengthened my faith in others.

— Rachel Haley: For being among the sweetest, most understanding people I first met in college, for showing a maturity few people possess, and for always supporting me and encouraging me to be my best self.

— Rick Cabagnot: For showing that the strong, seemingly silent type can cross boundaries and be the strong, understanding and incredibly kind type, and for being an unexpected source of strength and comfort throughout college.

— Jorge Quila, Jon White, Jeff Martinez, and Jerome Abedania: For being among the best college roommates and making the overall college experience that much more fun and accepting.

— Kiana Loftis (nee Humiston): For showing me what true loyalty and kindness is and for always being my partner in crime when we danced in our college workshops together.

— Marli Diestel: For being the best, most unselfish friend I have ever encountered, and for seeing and encouraging the potential and skill I possessed in all of the work we did in environmental social justice activism.

— Emma Hedermo: For showing me what passion, commitment, the beautiful effect of music, and the meaning of friendship and trust are all about.

— Elizabeth "Eli" Agustin: For showing such maturity at a young age, for telling me that honesty is the best quality I possess, and for never turning down any offer I made to spend time together.

— Mackenzie Conway: For showing that there are more sides to a person than are seen in first impressions, and in the process, becoming a trusted confidant and understanding human being.

— The Honorable Judge Harlan Grossman: For giving me the opportunity to explore and experience the inner workings of the justice system.

— The SFSU Divestment Campaign, Bill McKibben, and 350.org representatives: For giving me the opportunity of a lifetime to help create and be a part of a transformative movement that will define generations to come; special recognition to Evan Watson, Nick Cichetti, Michael Zambrano, Floreana Joelle Burila, Wade Vance, Jennifer Fong, Jason Schwartz, Alex Ansari, Rizzie Vermont,

Sara Blazevic, Theo LeQuense, Emily Williams, and Kevin Killion, to name a few. (The rest of you know who you are!)

— Sonya Soltani and Miguel Guerrero: For being forces to be reckoned with on the political front of our campaign and for being all around incredible friends and human beings.

— The SFSU International Student Community: For being one of the most inclusive groups of people I ever had the pleasure of getting to know; special recognition to Amelie de Rochfoucauld, Marie Lorraine, Alice Pinon, Farah Midani, Jun Kataoka, Jonnomei Colnot, Rie Tanaka, Ai Nakanishi, Jan Ster, and Kaiser Rangel!

— Patricia Akello: For being a true example of a strong individual in the face of unspeakable horrors; and for striving to make the world a better, more tolerant place; and for inspiring the activist in me.

— Kate Hallett: For taking advice I casually gave you and using it to transform an entire community in a way I never could have foreseen and of which I could not be prouder!

— Ariel Tyson: For showing me the definition of love and affection and that strong, mature people can make the best out of any situation.

— Jesse Kassner and Jacob Ritts: My FEMA brothers. Thank you for being by my side through all of the struggle and bringing out my fun side in bowling, laser tag, and Texas BBQ to make me feel normal and accepted!

— FEMA Region VI: For giving me such a comprehensive experience in the public sector workforce, with special recognition to Kelvin Mack and Laverm "Bullett" Young, Jr. for being great teachers, mentors, and above all, great human beings.

— Sundance Kabuki Cinema Managers Jennifer Tang and Jenny Vela for both allowing me to give my all to the cinema and being such strong and compassionate supporters in my mother's fight with cancer.

— Temarius Walker: For being my direct boss, eventual friend, and now honorary brother in all our future endeavors. You will change the world with your concept art and your unconditionally positive outlook in life that I wish I could aspire to have!

— Greg and Randy Gee: The two G's I cannot live without who are equal in compassion, charitable acts, and being fun-loving, authentic, and overall inspiring brothers I am beyond blessed to call my friends.

— Birthright Israel: For broadening my perspective and inspiring me to return to advance my career aspirations. Special recognition to Gal Nahmias, Amit Hameiri, Ziv Lehrman, Tomer Priel, Yael Barcessat, Guy Inbar, Alona Rahmani, Gary Lent and Rachelle Lent, Brie Frank, Sarah Shor, Marc Rosenberg, Ari Weiss, Zoe Goldberg, Hillary Menkowitz, Matt Wiener, Jon Stark, Sol Lichtman, Perry Rosenbaum, Evan Gooberman, and Jared Smith, to name a few.

— Ryan Eastham, Marcus Confino, and Ben Collins: For being the best, most awesome and relatable roommates, who made my home life and social experiences in Israel some of the most treasured memories I have.

— Yael "Ellie" Ben-Or: For being my best friend, greatest ally, and biggest challenger when it came to facing myself and seeing the best in me beyond my existing flaws during our time in Young Judaea.

— Antonia Ash-Ranger: For reminding me never to hold preconceived notions on anyone until I get to know them and shattering my expectations on what our relationship would become.

— Gili Angert: For being the pinnacle of what it means to be a selfless, committed, vulnerable individual, and above all, one of the most beautiful human beings I have ever met in my life; my experiences in Israel would never have been possible without you!

— The EcoPeace staff: For giving me the opportunity to work for an official nonprofit institution that had eluded me for so long; special recognition to Giulia Giordano, Gidon Bromberg, Rachel Weisbrot, Rotem Weizman, and Shlomit Tamari, to name a few.

— Masa Israel: For being the entire reason I was able to make a professional and personal life for myself in Israel and teaching me lessons I will never forget for the rest of my life; special recognition to Ben Baginsky, Josh Maya, Stephanie Jablon, Zach Richstone, Miranda Franklin-Wall, Roy Buchler, Asher Dale, Hannah Gerson, Shirly Said, Heather Hammerling, Annie Lashinsky, Irene Niskier,

Shayna Han, Tali Simon, Michael Tully, and Roni Rachmani, to name a few.

— The Tamari Family: For allowing me to feel like a part of a tight-knit, loving family and for including me in one of the holiest of Jewish celebrations; special recognition to Shlomit and Shir Tamari for making this happen.

— Young Judaea Spring Program participants and staff: For being the foundation and core of the entire experience and for showing me what it means to have an inclusive family that you can always count on when you need them; special recognition to Tamar Zer-Aviv and Dafna Meller for making the program and internships a reality for me; further recognition to Allan Binder, Ilan Renous, Allison Kekoler, Mollie Kesten, Danna Rosenfield, Johanna Scott, Rachel Rosenzweig, Cory Cassell, Alana Hayes, Willian Blanck, Ben Sotomayor, Valeriya "Lera" Nakshun, Mollie Teitelbaum, Marlee Rosenthal, Vasily Kronos, and Sara-Elizabeth Clark, to name a few.

And to all of the people I got to know through the various other environmental organizations, the district attorney's office, Hip Hop International, San Francisco State University, FEMA Region VI, the Dallas community, the Bay Area dance community, and the many friends and acquaintances I made during my stay in Israel, you all know who you are!

And finally to you, the reader, whether disabled or "normal," ordinary or extraordinary, a mother or father looking to be the best parent possible, or someone who wants a real, inspiring story to inspire you, my chapter ends here for another to begin elsewhere, and I hope this helps you begin a new chapter of your own. The story is now yours to create.

"Research your own experience, Absorb what is useful, Discard what is not, Add what is uniquely your own"

— Bruce Lee

ABOUT THE AUTHOR

Adam A.F. Sherman is a San Francisco-based writer and avid social justice activist. While continuing to struggle with anxiety and underdeveloped social skills, Adam has resolved to demonstrate to the world, and to future generations, that being limited does not mean staying limited. This is his first book.

ABOUT THE PUBLISHER

The Sager Group was founded in 1984. In 2012 it was chartered as a multimedia content brand, with the intent of empowering those who create art—an umbrella beneath which makers can pursue, and profit from, their craft directly, without gatekeepers. TSG publishes books; ministers to artists and provides modest grants; and produces documentary, feature, and commercial films. By harnessing the means of production, The Sager Group helps artists help themselves. For more information, please see www.TheSagerGroup.net.

MORE BOOKS FROM THE SAGER GROUP

The Swamp: Deceit and Corruption in the CIA
An Elizabeth Petrov Thriller (Book 1)
by Jeff Grant

Chains of Nobility: Brotherhood of the Mamluks (Book 1-3)
by Brad Graft

Meeting Mozart: A Novel Drawn from the Secret Diaries of Lorenzo Da Ponte
by Howard Jay Smith

Death Came Swiftly: A Novel About the Tay Bridge Disaster of 1879
by Bill Abrams

A Boy and His Dog in Hell: And Other Stories
by Mike Sager

Miss Havilland: A Novel
by Gay Daly

The Orphan's Daughter: A Novel
by Jan Cherubin

Lifeboat No. 8: Surviving the Titanic
by Elizabeth Kaye

Hunting Marlon Brando: A True Story by Mike Sager

See our entire library at TheSagerGroup.net

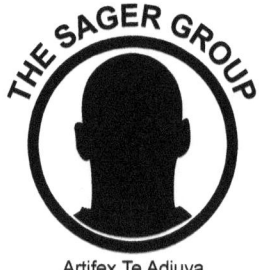

www.ingramcontent.com/pod-product-compliance
Lightning Source LLC
Chambersburg PA
CBHW030323100526
44592CB00010B/550